# CHALLENGING HEALTH INEQUALITIES

## From Acheson to 'Choosing health'

Edited by Elizabeth Dowler and Nick Spencer

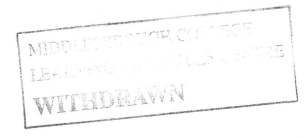

First published in Great Britain in 2007 by

The Policy Press
University of Bristol
Fourth Floor
Beacon House
Queen's Road
Bristol BS8 1QU
UK

Tel +44 (0)117 331 4054
Fax +44 (0)117 331 4093
e-mail tpp-info@bristol.ac.uk
www.policypress.org.uk

British Library Cataloguing in Publication Data
A catalogue record for this book is available from the British Library.

Library of Congress Cataloging-in-Publication Data
A catalog record for this book has been requested.

ISBN 978 1 86134 899 9 paperback
ISBN 978 1 86134 900 2 hardcover

Cover design by Qube Design Associates, Bristol.
Front cover: image kindly supplied by www.alamy.com
Printed and bound in Great Britain by MPG Books, Bodmin.

# Contents

# List of tables and figures

## Tables

## Figures

# Acknowledgements

The idea for this volume arose out of the experience of a conference at Warwick in December 2003 hosted, at Sir Donald Acheson's suggestion, by the Institute of Health: The Acheson Inquiry: Five Years On. Nick Spencer and Elizabeth Dowler would like to thank the co-directors of the Institute of Health at Warwick, Professor Gillian Hundt and Dr Hannah Bradby, for their encouragement and support in the editing of the book. Simon Williams, Michael Calnan and Alan Dolan would like to thank Richard Wilkinson, Gareth Williams and Graham Scambler for their valuable contributions to the conference workshop entitled 'Explaining inequalities in health', from which their chapter is, in part, derived.

# Notes on contributors

**Peter Beresford** is Professor of Social Policy and Director of the Centre for Citizen Participation at Brunel University. He is also Chair of Shaping Our Lives, the independent national service user controlled organisation and network, a trustee of the Social Care Institute for Excellence, and Visiting Fellow at the School for Social Work and Psychsocial Studies at University of East Anglia. He has a particular interest in issues of participation and participatory research.

**Hannah Bradby** is Associate Professor in the Department of Sociology, at the University of Warwick, specialising in the sociology of health and sociology of ethnicity. Recent articles include '"Watch out for the Aunties":Young British Asians' accounts of identity and substance use', *Sociology of Health and Illness* (in press); and (with R. Williams),'Is religion or culture the key feature in changes in substance use after leaving school? Asians and non-Asians in Glasgow', (2006) *Ethnicity and Health*, vol 1, no 3, pp 307-24.

**Paul Bywaters** is Emeritus Professor of Social Work, Coventry University, and Honorary Professor at the University of Warwick. He jointly founded the international Social Work and Health Inequalities Network (www.warwick.ac.uk/go/swhin) of which he was Convenor until the end of 2006. His publications include P. Bywaters and E.McLeod (eds), *Working for equality in health* (Routledge, 1996); E. McLeod and P. Bywaters, *Social work, health and equality* (Routledge, 2000); and G. Letherby and P. Bywaters, *Extending social research* (Open University Press, 2006).

**Michael Calnan** is Professor of Medical Sociology at the University of Kent. He has worked in health policy and services research and training for over 20 years, his most recent previous post being Professor of Medical Sociology in the Medical Research Council Health Services Research Collaboration, in the Department of Social Medicine, University of Bristol. Current research interests include: diffusion and innovation in health care and technology, comparative health care systems, trust in healthcare and ageing, and health and social care, and he has published extensively in this field.

**Martin Caraher** is Reader in Food and Health Policy, Department of Health Management and Food Policy, Institute of Health Sciences, City University, London. His main interests are in the areas of food poverty, cooking skills, local sustainable food supplies, the role of markets and co-ops in promoting health, food deserts and food access, retail concentration and globalisation. He sits on the London Food Board, advising the Mayor of London, and the South East Food and Public Health Group. Recent publications include T. Lang and M. Caraher, 'Global public health', in D. Pencheon et al, *Oxford handbook of public health practice* (Oxford University Press, 2006); and M. Caraher et al, 'TV advertising and children: Lessons from policy development' (2006) *Public Health Nutrition*, vol 9, no 5, pp 596–605.

**Mick Carpenter** is Reader in Social Policy, Department of Sociology, University of Warwick, whose research interests include regeneration and community development, participative approaches to evaluation, inequalities in health, labour market issues, and health and social policy. He is co-author (with S. Jefferys) of *Management, work and welfare in Western Europe* (Edward Elgar, 2000). Recent publications include 'The health of nations: What the Greek case tells us about the social determinants of health', in *Social Policy Review 15* (The Policy Press, 2003), pp 111-31.

**Tarani Chandola** is Senior Lecturer in Medical Sociology in the Department of Epidemiology and Public Health, University College London. His work includes research on the measurement of social position in relation to health, explaining social, ethnic and geographical variations in health and analysing the role of psychosocial factors in explaining social inequalities in health. He has recently published Chandola et al, 'Pathways between education and health: a causal modelling approach'(2006) *Journal of the Royal Statistics Society*, Series A, vol 169, no 2, pp 337-59; and Chandola et al, 'Chronic stress at work and the metabolic syndrome: prospective study' (2006) *BMJ*, vol 332, pp 521-5.

**Suzy Croft** is Research Fellow at Brunel University, and a senior social worker at St John's Hospice, London. She is a member of the editorial collective of *Critical Social Policy*. She has particular interests in participation and palliative care, and is a former Chair of the Association of Palliative Care Social Workers. Her most recent publications include

P. Beresford, L. Adshead and S. Croft, *Palliative care, social work and service users* (Jessica Kingsley, 2006).

**George Davey Smith** is Professor of Clinical Epidemiology at the University of Bristol, Scientific Director of the Avon Longitudinal Study of Parents and their Children (ALSPAC) and Director of the MRC Centre for Causal Analyses in Translational Epidemiology. His research interests centre on lifecourse influences on health inequalities;, genetic epidemiology and epidemiological methodology. His publications include *Health inequalities: Lifecourse approaches* (The Policy Press, 2003) and he is editor of the *International Journal of Epidemiology*.

**Alan Dolan** is Associate Professor in Health and Social Policy, Institute of Health, School of Health and Social Studies, University of Warwick. His research interests lie in inequalities in health, men's health, fatherhood, poverty and smoking, and current and forthcoming publications include Dolan et al, '"You ain't going to say … I've got a problem down there": workplace-based prostate health promotion with men' (2005) *Health Education Research: Theory and Practice*, vol 20, no 6, pp 730-8, and '"Good luck to them if they can get it": Exploring working class men's understandings and experiences of income inequality and material standards' (2007) *Sociology of Health and Illness* vol 29, no 5, pp 1-19.

**Danny Dorling** is Professor of Human Geography, Department of Geography, University of Sheffield. He has previously worked in Bristol and Leeds, and now works on a project to remap the world (www.worldmapper.com). His research interests include social and spatial inequalities, and improving the understanding of patterns to people's lives by cartography and statistics. Recent publications include (with B. Thomas) *Identity in Britain: A cradle-to-grave atlas* (The Policy Press, 2007) and (with many colleagues) *Poverty, wealth and place in Britain, 1968-2005* (The Policy Press, 2007).

**Elizabeth Dowler** is Reader in Food and Social Policy, Department of Sociology, University of Warwick. Her research interests are in poverty, food, nutrition and public health, particularly for families; evaluating food/nutrition policy and local initiatives; people's views of risk in food; and the benefits of 'alternative' food networks. She is a member of the Food Ethics Council, and the Programme Development Group for Maternal and Child Nutrition Public Health Programme Guidance for

NICE. Recent publications include E. Dowler and C. Jones Finer (eds) *The welfare of food: Rights and responsibilities in a changing world* (Blackwells, 2003); P. Mosley and E. Dowler (eds), *Poverty and social exclusion in North and South* (Routledge, 2003); Dowler et al, *Poverty bites: Food, health and poor families* (Child Poverty Action Group, 2001).

**Mark Drakeford** is Professor of Social Policy and Applied Social Sciences at the University of Wales, Cardiff. He currently works as the Cabinet health and social policy adviser, and special adviser to the First Minister at the Welsh Assembly Government. He has published extensively on social work, social policy and poverty, his most recent publications including *Privatisation and social policy* (Longman, 2000) and (with I. Butler) *Scandal, social policy and social welfare* (The Policy Press, 2005).

**Ray Earwicker** is a senior member of the Health Inequalities Unit, in the Department of Health. He was secretary to the Independent Inquiry into Inequalities in Health, chaired by Sir Donald Acheson in 1998.

**Catherine Law** is Reader in Children's Health and Director of the Centre for Policy Research at the Centre for Paediatric Epidemiology and Biostatistics, University College London Institute of Child Health. Her research interests lie in paediatric epidemiology and child public health, particularly the development of cardiovascular risk factors in children, physical growth, and inequalities in child health. Her published articles include 'Significance of birth weight for the future' (2002) *Archives of Disease in Childhood, Fetal Neonatal Edition*, vol 86, no 1, pp F7-F8, and, as co-author, 'Body size at birth and blood pressure among children in developing countries' (2001) *International Journal of Epidemiology* February, vol 30, no 1, pp 52-7, and 'A systematic review of lay views about infant size and growth' (2006) *Archives of Disease in Childhood*, August 11.

**Helen Lester** is Professor of Primary Care at the National Centre for Primary Care Research and Development, University of Manchester. She is national primary care lead for the Mental Health Research Network, and Academic Lead of the Expert Panel reviewing the GP Contract Quality and Outcomes Framework. She was a GP in inner city Birmingham for 17 years. She has written over 90 papers, chapters and books, most focused on mental health policy and practice, health inequalities, service user involvement and, more recently, health outcome measurement.

**Paul Lincoln** is Chief Executive of the National Heart Forum, based in London. He is also Director of the WHO Collaborating Centre Programme (HEA) on investment in health and health promotion; a consultant/advisor to WHO, the European Commission, the WHO Countrywide Integrated Non-communicable Diseases Intervention (CINDI) programme, and to various governments on health promotion. He has been involved in the establishment and management of the European Network of National Health Promotion/Public Health Agencies, and is a member of the WHO Health Promotion Evaluation Policy-Experts group and Chair of the European Health Forum Advisory Committee/European Heart Network.

**Eileen McLeod** is Associate Professor (Reader) at the School of Health and Social Studies, University of Warwick. Her research interests centre on social work's contribution to tackling health inequalities and she has published extensively in this area. She is a founder member of SWHIN (Social Work and Health Inequalities Network), the first international network of social work researchers and practitioners addressing health inequalities. Her publications include E. McLeod and P Bywaters, *Social work, health and equality* (Routledge, 2000).

**David Ormandy** is Principal Research Fellow and Director of the Safe and Health Housing Research Unit at the Department of Law, University of Warwick. He specialises in the formulation of standards and the relationship between environment (particularly housing environment) and health, and has worked with WHO European Centre for Environment and Health on housing and health matters including accidental home injuries, indoor air quality, and the development of Environmental Health Indicators. He is the project manager responsible to the Office of the Deputy Prime Minister for the development of the Housing Health and Safety Rating System (from April 2006 the statutory prescribed method for the assessment of housing conditions in England).

**Mary Shaw** is Scientific Director of the South West Public Health Observatory and Reader in Medical Sociology, Department of Social Medicine, University of Bristol. Her interests lie in social and geographical inequalities in mortality and morbidity, social and spatial accumulation of health inequalities, poverty and health of disadvantaged groups (particularly homeless people), health and social policies, and photography in social science. Her publications include M. Shaw, D. Dorling and R. Mitchell, *Health, place and society* (Pearson, 2002), G. Davey Smith and M. Shaw (eds), *Cultures of health, cultures of illness*, British Medical Bulletin (Oxford University Press, 2004) and (with B. Wheeler, R. Mitchell and D. Dorling) *Life in Britain: Using Millennial Census data to understand poverty, inequality and place* (The Policy Press, 2005).

**Nick Spencer** is Professor Emeritus of Child Health, School of Health and Social Studies, University of Warwick, with research interests in poverty and child health, child health inequalities, and the social determinants of health across the early lifecourse. He is author of *Weighing the evidence: How is birthweight determined?* (Radcliffe Press, 2003), and articles including: Spencer et al, 'Disabling conditions and child abuse and neglect: a population-based study', (2005) *Pediatrics* vol 116, pp 609-13; 'Maternal education, lone parenthood, material hardship, maternal smoking and longstanding respiratory problems in childhood: Testing a hierarchical conceptual framework' (2005) *Journal of Epidemiology and Community Health*, vol 59, pp 842-6; and 'Explaining the social gradient in smoking in pregnancy' (2006) *Social Science and Medicine*, vol 62, pp 1250-9.

**Jonathan Tritter** is Chief Executive of the NHS Centre for Involvement, and Professorial Fellow in the Institute of Governance and Public Management, Warwick Business School, University of Warwick. The NHS Centre for Involvement was established to work with NHS staff and their organisations to engage with patients and the public more effectively. His particular area of interest is public participation and lay experience in health and policy making, especially in relation to cancer, mental health and environmental policy. His publications include Anderson, Tritter and Wilsons (eds), *Healthy democracy: Involving people in health and social care* (INVOLVE, 2006); Tritter et al, *Improving cancer services through user involvement* (Radcliffe Medical Press, 2003); H. Lester, J. Tritter and H. Sorohan, 'Providing "good enough" primary care for people with serious mental illness – a focus group study' (2005) *British Medical Journal*, vol 330, pp 1122-7; and J. Tritter and A. McCallum, 'The snakes and ladders of user involvement: Moving beyond Arnstein' (2006) *Health Policy*, vol 76, no 2, pp 156-68.

**Simon J. Williams** is Professor of Sociology at the University of Warwick, with research interests in the sociology of health. His current research centres on the pharmaceutical industry. He has published extensively in medical sociology and related domains, including ten books and contributions to leading journals in the field ,such as *Sociology of Health and Illness, Social Science and Medicine, Health,* and *The International Journal of Health Services.*

# ONE

# Introduction

## Nick Spencer and Elizabeth Dowler

New Labour has been in government in the UK for almost 10 years. From early in its period of office, it set out to challenge the official indifference to the public health significance of health inequalities. Within six months of taking office, the Acheson Inquiry into inequalities in health was convened with the remit of recommending policies aimed at reducing health inequalities. The inquiry report was published in 1998 by the Department of Health for England and Wales (Acheson, 1998)..It is timely to take stock of progress in reducing what the report describes as 'unacceptable inequalities in health' and assess the extent to which the report's recommendations have been enacted by government up to and including the public health White Paper (DH, 2004). This book draws on the work of authors from various disciplines to explore the extent to which New Labour policy since taking office advances the policy agenda recommended by the Acheson Inquiry. The book presents the perspectives of different disciplines, some of which, though engaged with health inequalities, are rarely heard in the policy and practice debates. Of necessity, the book's main focus is England; however, where appropriate, authors draw on policy initiatives in the other nations of the UK. Although touching on many similar areas to recent books by Exworthy et al (2003) addressing progress in tackling health inequalities since Acheson, and Asthana and Halliday (2006) addressing what works in tackling health inequalities, the book has a different focus and approaches the challenge of health inequalities from a different perspective. Policy areas that are major drivers of health inequalities, such as poverty, income distribution, education and employment, are considered within chapters (for example, in Chapters Three and Five) rather than as separate subject areas.

## The importance and extent of health inequalities

Avoidable inequalities in health experience and outcomes related to socioeconomic status at individual, household or area level, ethnicity and gender have been identified at all stages of the life course from pregnancy to old age. Such inequalities make a major contribution to avoidable mortality and ill health. These issues are widely documented in the literature and, recently, in government policy statements. For example, based on studies in the West Midlands region of England (Spencer et al, 1999a) and the city of Sheffield (Spencer et al, 1999b), the proportion of infants with low birth-weight (<2,500 g) and very low birth-weight (<1,500 g) would be reduced by 30% and 32% respectively if all infants had the same birth-weight distribution as those in the most privileged tenth of the population. Low birth-weight is itself an indicator of present and future risk of ill health and reduced capacity (Paneth, 1995; Barker, 1998; Spencer, 2003).

The impact of inequalities in health in adulthood is reflected in the fact that three quarters of the premature (that is, pre-65 years of age) adult deaths that occur in the deprived area of Glasgow known as Shettleston would not occur if Shettleston had the same mortality rates as the privileged area of Wokingham (Shaw et al, 1999). The striking differences in life expectancy between electoral wards within the same London boroughs are shown in Table 1.1, taken from the UK government's public health White Paper *Choosing health: Making healthier choices easier* (DH, 2004).

Although the prevalence and extent of inequalities depends on the outcome studied, the overall effect of inequalities on population health is considerable and their reduction is key both to equity in health and to overall population health gain.

**Table 1.1: Life expectancy differences within selected London boroughs**

| Borough | Lowest ward level life expectancy | Highest ward level life expectancy | Difference (years) |
|---|---|---|---|
| Westminster male | 67.4 | 82.6 | 15.2 |
| Westminster female | 72.2 | 86.4 | 14.2 |
| Camden male | 69.5 | 79.6 | 10.1 |
| Camden female | 76.4 | 87.1 | 10.7 |

*Source:* DH (2004, p 83)

# From the Black Report to the Acheson Inquiry: revival of interest in health inequalities

The report of the Acheson Inquiry was published 18 years after the so-called Black Report (from the name of the chair of the working party, Sir Douglas Black), which had been commissioned by the previous Labour government, but which was not published until 1980, by which time Labour had lost the election in 1979. The incoming Conservative administration was hostile to the recommendations of the Black Report and tried to limit publication. It was subsequently published as a book (Townsend and Davidson, 1982), which is its most familiar and accessible form. Despite its troubled origins, the Black Report became a highly influential publication nationally and internationally. It revived interest in the social determinants of health, engendered lively theoretical debate and practical research, and presented evidence to support structural explanations for inequalities in health (Davey Smith et al, 1990a). Its history and effects have been debated and widely discussed (for example, Berridge and Blume, 2003).

In the 18 years between the publication of the two reports, there was an explosion of published literature related to health inequalities, exploring both their extent and the mechanisms generating them. This upsurge in research took place in the face of attempts by the UK and US governments to discourage research into the structural influences on health and their insistence that health inequalities be characterised as 'health variations'. Having initially focused on describing inequalities, research interest shifted to look at trends (Shaw et al, 1999) and the mechanisms generating and sustaining health inequalities (Davey Smith et al, 1990b, among many).

Against a background of improving health across the whole population, evidence emerged of widening health inequalities associated with slower health gains among the most disadvantaged compared with the most privileged (see, for example, McLoone and Boddy, 1994; Shaw et al, 1999). As Shaw et al (1999) suggested, these trends were related to the dramatic increases in poverty and deprivation that were part of the legacy of 18 years of Conservative government. Research into the mechanisms by which health inequalities are generated and sustained followed various lines of enquiry. The newly emergent field of life-course epidemiology (Kuh and Ben-Shlomo, 1997) owed its origins in large part to studies that identified links between poor childhood social circumstances and increased risk of mortality due to coronary artery disease in adult life (for example, Forsdahl, 1977). Further work, demonstrating the relationship of fetal and early childhood social circumstances to a range of later health outcomes (see, for example, Power et al, 1991; Barker, 1992), confirmed that health inequalities could not be understood solely in relation to current social circumstances; rather, explanations had to take account of social risk exposures over the life course.

Interest also centred on the role of ethnicity and the experience of minority ethnic populations in generating health inequalities (see, for example, Williams, 1992; Benzeval et al, 1995; Harding and Balarajan, 2000). It was clear that many minority ethnic groups had poorer health outcomes than the majority population and much, but not all, of this disparity was explained by the relative socioeconomic disadvantage of these groups (Nazroo, 2003). Thus, these groups were noted to experience 'double jeopardy' – the effects on health of disadvantage plus the effects of discrimination and racism. Children and adults with disabilities were also shown to experience 'double jeopardy' due to a combination of material disadvantage and discrimination, particularly in the job market (Hogan et al, 1997; Jenkins and Rigg, 2003).

Socioeconomic factors such as income and education do not exert a direct effect on health leading to health inequalities. Their effects are mediated through other variables acting singly or together to influence health. Health-related behaviour is the mediator that has generated most interest. Although explanations for health inequalities (or 'variations' as they were called) based on choice and individual behaviour dominated official publications and policy statements prior to 1997 (DH, 1992, 1996), researchers began to explore the relationship between adverse health-related behaviours, particularly smoking, and material disadvantage (Graham, 1994; Power and Matthews, 1997). Poor nutrition, which had been characterised by Conservative minister, Ann Widdecombe, during an interview on BBC Radio 4's Today programme in 1991 as the result of failure to shop carefully enough, was also shown to be intimately linked with material disadvantage and a key mediator of health inequalities (see, for example, NCH, 1991; Dowler and Calvert, 1995; Lobstein, 1997). Housing (see, for example, Lowry, 1991; Ineichen, 1993), work (see, for example, Marmot et al, 1997; Power and Matthews, 1997) and stress (see, for example, Brunner, 1997) were studied as other potential mediators of the relationship between social status and health.

## Social gradients in health: the emergence of different explanations

The renewed interest in health inequalities prompted by the Black Report opened up a debate on explanations for social gradients in health. The finely graded relationship between some health outcomes and socioeconomic status across the spectrum demonstrated that, for these outcomes at least, increased risk compared with the most advantaged was not confined to the most disadvantaged, but affected the moderately advantaged as well (Davey Smith et al, 1990b; Marmot, 2004). Attempts to explain social gradients produced broadly two schools of thought: adverse health effects were produced by the stress of perceived unfairness associated with subordinate positions in the social hierarchy (Wilkinson, 1996; Marmot, 2004), or were the effects of socially patterned risk factors accumulating longitudinally and clustering cross-sectionally (Bartley et al, 1997; Berney et al, 2000). The former drew partly on animal studies (Sameroff and Suomi, 1996), and on the increasing interest in the association of income inequality with variation in the health of populations (Kennedy et al, 1996; Wilkinson, 1996). The latter drew on life-course epidemiology (Kuh and Ben-Shlomo, 1997), particularly the association between early childhood socioeconomic status and adult health (Berney et al, 2000).

Nonetheless, there is broad agreement between these schools of thought that health inequalities based on social position are unjust, requiring policy measures to reduce them; however, because of their differing theoretical perspectives, their policy solutions can be widely divergent. One school of thought lays particular emphasis on enhancing social capital as a means of counteracting perceived unfairness and the psychological consequences of inequality (for example, Kawachi et al, 1997). The other school advocates materialist solutions to the problems of poverty and poor social circumstances (for example, Lynch et al, 2000). The debate on these differing explanations of health inequalities is ongoing and is reflected later in this book. Chapter Three is a critique New Labour policy from a clear materialist perspective, while Chapter Four suggests that structural changes in material circumstances are essential to reducing health inequalities and that the psychosocial school is, in fact, a refinement of the materialist school. Chapter Eleven further explores these issues, highlighting the tension between 'bottom-up' approaches that seek to increase local 'social capital' and 'top-down' approaches that ignore the local context.

Notwithstanding the conclusions of Black and Acheson that structural explanations for inequalities in health are powerfully supported by the evidence and have to be a key focus for potential intervention, in practice a third school of thought has continued to favour health 'behaviour and lifestyle' explanations for health inequalities. Thus, inequalities in a range of adverse outcomes such as birth-weight (Bonellie, 2001), sudden infant death (Blair et al, 1996) and cardiovascular disease mortality (Strand and Tverdal, 2004) are explained primarily in terms of individual behaviours and so-called 'lifestyle' choices, where these are seen as largely determined by the decision making and under the control of the individual. Policies flowing from this school of thought centre on changing such health-related behaviours as though they were mainly open to individual choice, and independent from any structural inequalities underpinning them.

## The significance of the Acheson Inquiry and its recommendations

On coming to power in 1997, one of New Labour's election commitments was to end inequalities in health. The Acheson Inquiry, therefore, in contrast to the working party chaired by Sir Douglas Black, carried out its work in a period when academic research and practitioner support for health inequalities was high and the political climate appeared conducive to bringing about change. The new government had opened up public discourse on health inequalities and had committed itself to an evidence-based policy approach to reduce inequalities. The inquiry team, consisting of Professor Sir Donald Acheson (chair), Professor David Barker, Dr Jacky Chambers, Professor Hilary Graham, Professor Sir Michael Marmot and Professor Margaret Whitehead, drew on scientific and expert evidence, and peer review, to identify areas for policy development likely to reduce inequalities in health. Like the authors of the Black Report, they concluded that the weight of evidence supports a socioeconomic explanation for health inequalities, rather than one rooted in individual choice. They thus traced the roots of ill health to determinants such as income, education and employment as well as to the material environment and lifestyle.

Such a conclusion led them to make recommendations across the whole of government policy, with implications for all departments, not just the Department of Health. There were two general recommendations and 37 recommendations related to specific policy areas. The first general recommendation stated that, as part of health impact assessment, all policies likely to have a direct or indirect effect on health should be evaluated in terms of their impact on health inequalities and, furthermore, should be formulated in such a way that by favouring the less well off they will, wherever possible, reduce such inequalities. The second general recommendation was that high priority should be given to policies aimed at improving health, and reducing health inequalities, in women of childbearing age, expectant mothers and young children. The remaining recommendations covered the areas of poverty, income, tax and benefits; education; employment; housing and environment; mobility, transport and pollution; nutrition and the Common Agricultural Policy; mothers, children and families; young people and adults of working age; older people; ethnicity; gender; and the National Health Service.

The recommendations of particular relevance to subject areas covered in this book – housing, nutrition, mothers, children and families, and ethnicity – are examined in the relevant chapters. However, it is useful to outline them briefly here in order to position the chapters dealing with specific areas in relation to the inquiry and subsequent policy.

In relation to housing and the environment, the inquiry made four recommendations (recommendations 10-13): improved availability of social housing with a framework of environmental improvement, planning and design; improved housing provision for homeless people; improved housing quality specifically in relation to insulation and heating, regulations on space and amenities; policies aimed at reducing the fear of crime and violence, and creating safe living environments. One recommendation specifically dealt with nutrition and its role in health inequalities (recommendation 20): policies that will increase the availability and accessibility of foodstuffs to supply an adequate and affordable diet, specifically those policies that will ensure adequate retail provision of food to those who are disadvantaged.

Three specific recommendations flowed from the inquiry's second general recommendation that high priority be given to policies aimed at reducing inequalities among mothers and children (recommendations 21-23): policies that reduce poverty in families with children by promoting the material support of parents, by removing barriers to work for parents who wish to combine work with parenting and by enabling those who wish to devote themselves full time to parenting to do so; policies that improve the health and nutrition of women of childbearing age and their children, with priority given to the elimination of food poverty and the prevention and reduction of obesity; policies that promote the social and emotional support for parents and children.

The inquiry addressed the 'double jeopardy' of minority ethnic populations with the following recommendations (recommendations 31-33): specific consideration of the needs of minority ethnic groups in the development and implementation of policies aimed at reducing socioeconomic inequalities; the further development of services that are sensitive to the needs of minority ethnic people and promote greater awareness of their health risks; specific consideration of the needs of minority ethnic groups in needs assessment, resource allocation, healthcare planning and provision.

Although criticised as 'too vague to be useful' (Davey Smith et al, 1998), the recommendations in practice represented a radical departure from the policy directions of the previous government, as well as providing a policy template on which the New Labour government could build its measures to reduce inequalities in health. Thus, coming as they did at the beginning of the new government's term of office, the recommendations had the potential to influence policy directions and make a positive contribution to reducing the injustice of health inequalities. This book aims to examine the recommendations of the Acheson Inquiry within the policy framework of the New Labour administration enacted in the 10 years since its election, assess the extent to which policy has followed Acheson's recommendations, and discuss the effects they have had on inequalities in health.

## Inequalities and recent policy initiatives

It is not our intention in this introductory chapter to present an exhaustive overview of policy initiatives designed to reduce health inequalities. These issues are addressed in detail in the following chapters. However, it seems appropriate to mention briefly some key initiatives relevant to the theme of the book, since its overall aim is to assess their effectiveness in reducing health inequalities. Government activities to tackle health inequalities have been generated from a range of departments, led or supported by, or in collaboration with, the Department of Health, although from the outset, the department has emphasised the need for a 'partnership' approach: that government and individuals each have responsibilities and a part to play in reducing health inequalities. In its report *Tackling health inequalities: A Programme for Action* (DH, 2003), the Department of Health laid claim to 62 new initiatives on inequalities and, for the first time, established targets for reductions in specific health inequalities. The second of the Acheson Inquiry general recommendations has been followed in so far as a range of programmes aimed at overcoming disadvantage in early childhood has been set up. These include Sure Start, plans to increase access to early childhood education, and working family tax credits.

Other listed policy initiatives that relate to specific areas highlighted by the Acheson Inquiry include tax credits and the minimum wage to address low income; the New Deal to reduce long-term unemployment; plans to ensure nursery places for all three-year-olds; and the Free Fruit in Schools programme. The implementation of these and other initiatives, and whether they have been effective in reducing health inequalities, is the subject of much debate and is discussed in the chapters that follow

As part of the review of the costs of ill health to the nation, the Treasury commissioned a report from Derek Wanless (2002), a merchant banker, into the resource implications of providing high-quality services and catching up with other developed countries in terms of health and well-being. The report identified considerable differences in expected costs depending both on the improved performance of the health services and on how well the population became fully engaged with its own health. In 2004, the Treasury commissioned a second report, *Securing good health for the whole population* (Wanless, 2004), which focused on prevention and wider health determinants in England. The report concludes:

> Individuals are ultimately responsible for their own and their children's health and it is the aggregate actions of individuals, which will ultimately be responsible for whether or not such an optimistic scenario as 'fully engaged' unfolds. People need to be supported more actively to make better decisions about their own health and welfare because there are widespread, systematic failures that influence the decisions individuals currently make. (Wanless, 2004, p 4)

Informed by the conclusions of the Wanless Report (2004) and a wide public consultation, the government published its public health White Paper for England (DH, 2004), a key objective of which is to reduce health inequalities. The White Paper, *Choosing health: Making healthier choices easier* (DH, 2004), as its title suggests, focuses on enabling everyone to choose healthy lifestyles as its mechanism for improving public health and addressing health inequalities. Indeed, health inequalities are seen as the cumulative results of thousands of choices over long periods, thus prompting policy responses that seek to make healthy choices easier:

> Our fundamental aim must be to create a society where more people, particularly those in disadvantaged groups or areas, are encouraged and enabled to make healthier choices.

> In order to close the gap, we must ensure that the most
> marginalised and excluded groups and areas in society see
> faster improvements in health. (DH, 2004, p 11)

The implications of this apparent shift towards a 'choice' agenda and
to individual responsibility for health, as represented by the White
Paper as a means of achieving reductions in health inequalities, are
discussed in the chapters that follow, in relation to specific aspects of
health inequalities and their determinants.

## The widening gap

Despite New Labour's commitment to reducing health inequalities
and the plethora of initiatives and publications, social disparities in
health outcomes in England widened in the period 2001-03 compared
with 1997-99 (Dyer, 2005). Against two national health inequalities
targets announced in 2001, the gap between the poorest and the rest
of the population has widened. The gap in life expectancy between the
areas with the worst health and deprivation indicators (known as the
'spearhead group') and the population as a whole, targeted to reduce
by 10% by 2010, increased for the period 2001-03 compared with
1997-99. For males, the relative gap increased by nearly 2%, and for
females by 5% (DH, 2005). The gap in infant mortality rates between
'routine and manual' groups and the population as a whole, targeted
to reduce by 10% by 2010, also increased for the period 2001-03
compared with 1997-99.

Responses to this evidence of a widening gap varied. Rod Griffiths,
president of the Faculty of Public Health, quoted by Dyer (2005, p 419),
said the efforts undertaken so far showed that 'the government's heart
is in the right place on this issue but the task is a monumental one,
and there's no certainty that they can turn around a longstanding social
trend'. Michael Marmot, chairman of the scientific research group that
authored the report, also quoted by Dyer (2005), indicated that the
findings on life expectancy came as no surprise to his group but they
did note social changes that might be expected to have an effect on
health in years to come, of which the biggest was a dramatic reduction
in the number of children in poverty. The Minister for Public Health,
in a foreword to the DH document (DH, 2005, p 1), acknowledges the
widening gap, but states that 'there are, however, signs that some of the
indicators associated with health inequalities are moving in the right
direction. The progress achieved in tackling and seriously reducing child
poverty will contribute to reducing health inequalities in the future'.

Shaw et al (2005), in a letter to the *British Medical Journal*, linked the lack of progress on targets to the widening inequalities in income and wealth that had continued under the New Labour administration.

Against this background of widening inequalities despite policy initiatives and continuing government commitment to reducing health inequalities, it is timely to review progress in tackling health inequalities from the vantage point of different disciplines and subject areas and explore the extent to which current policy directions are likely to achieve the targets the government has set. That is what this book sets out to do.

## Structure and content of the book

This book differs from many that have addressed health inequalities in that it focuses on the strategies adopted by a government that set out specifically to reduce health inequalities, critically examining policies and programmes introduced during its first 10 years in office.

As previously mentioned, the book gives voice to disciplinary perspectives that, while pertinent to the health inequalities debate, are rarely heard. For example, Chapter Seven discusses housing policy and health inequalities from a legal perspective; Chapter Ten explores policy related to public participation and its impact on health inequalities; and Chapter Twelve considers a new agenda for social work in addressing health inequalities. As the book encompasses multiple perspectives, there are inevitably differences of emphasis and divergences of view on the effectiveness of current policies between authors. Broadly, chapter authors subscribe to the structural/materialist explanation of health inequalities and view 'Choosing health' as a reversion to discredited behavioural explanations that foster policy strategies based on individual rather than societal responsibility for health. Chapters Ten to Twelve examine the extent to which the voluntary sector, healthcare users and local activists have enabling roles in challenging health inequalities.

Chapters are broadly organised into four groups: overviews of policy, progress and theory in challenging health inequalities; determinants of inequality; factors that mediate those determinants; and sectoral policy interests. Three overview chapters give differing views on policy and progress since the Acheson Inquiry: Ray Earwicker (Chapter Two), a Department of Health policy maker involved in the Acheson Inquiry, discusses its impact on subsequent policy and the challenge of maintaining an effective focus on inequalities; Chapter Three presents a trenchant materialist critique of progress based on widening inequalities in mortality rates; and Chapter Four examines developments in theoretical and methodological issues that underpin policy strategies aimed at reducing health inequalities.

Two key determinants of health throughout the life course – experiences in pregnancy and early childhood, and ethnicity – are considered in the following two chapters. Chapter Five critically assesses the impact of the numerous New Labour policy initiatives aimed at reducing disadvantage in early childhood and reducing the effects of adverse early life experience on health inequalities across the life course. Chapter Six considers the evidence relating to ethnicity and health inequalities, identifying the compounding effects of poorer social circumstances and racism on minority ethnic groups and discussing the policy implications.

The next three chapters focus on important mediators of the relationship between social conditions and health. Chapter Seven tackles the impact of housing conditions on health inequalities, reviewing changes in legislation and experience since the report of the findings of the Acheson Inquiry (Acheson, 1998). Chapter Eight examines the role of food and nutrition, and the rapidly changing pressures and policy initiatives that potentially address inequalities. Chapter Nine summarises theoretical issues and contemporary practice in behavioural change, using cigarette smoking as a case study.

Specific policy initiatives in different sectors are examined in the next three chapters, in each case with evaluation of their impact on inequalities. Participation, consumer choice and empowerment are particularly important policy drivers under New Labour, as elsewhere. Chapter Ten examines the theory and practice of 'user involvement' and its impact on inequalities and Chapter Eleven examines the history and contemporary experience of local action and community development. Finally, drawing on a range of professional experiences, Chapter Twelve considers the new agenda for social work in addressing inequalities in physical health since the report of the findings of the Acheson Inquiry (Acheson, 1998). A concluding chapter draws together the main unifying themes and highlights further research, policy and practice challenges if health inequalities are to be significantly reduced.

The rhetoric about tackling inequalities in health is widely known and classical risk factor interventions are being implemented and evaluated under various circumstances. This is laudable. However, the limitations of such approaches are also widely acknowledged, especially where these risk factors (on diet and smoking, for instance) are seen as under individual control and there is potential for change (see, for example, Hunter, 2005). The wider public health agenda has to engage with structural, environmental issues, in both understanding health determinants and in constructing workable policy interventions. Nowhere is this more challenging than in reducing inequalities in health experience and outcomes. In bringing together a wide range of professional and academic experiences, this book contributes to addressing the critical upstream issues in contemporary societies.

## References

Acheson, D. (1998) *Independent inquiry into inequalities in health*, London: The Stationery Office.

Asthana, S. and Halliday, J. (2006) *What works in tackling health inequalities? Pathways, policies and practice through the lifecourse*, Bristol: The Policy Press.

Barker, D.J.P. (1992) *Fetal and infant origins of adult disease*, London: BMJ Publications Group.

Barker, D.J.P. (1998) *Mothers, babies and disease in later life* (2nd edn), Edinburgh: Churchill Livingstone.

Bartley, M., Blane, D. and Montgomery, S. (1997) 'Health and the life course: why safety nets matter', *BMJ*, vol 314, pp 1194-9.

Benzeval, M., Judge, K. and Smaje, C. (1995) 'Beyond class, race, and ethnicity: deprivation and health in Britain', *Health Services Research*, vol 30, no 1, pt 2, pp 163-77.

Berney, L., Blane, D., Davey Smith, G. and Holland, P. (2000) 'Lifecourse influences on health in early old age', in H. Graham (ed) *Understanding health inequalities*, Buckingham: Open University Press, pp 79-95.

Berridge, V. and Blume, S. (2003) *Poor health. Social inequality before and after the Black Report*, London: Frank Cass.

Blair, P.S., Fleming, P.J., Bensley, D., Smith, I., Bacon, C., Taylor, E., Berry, J., Golding, J. and Tripp, J. (1996) 'Smoking and the sudden infant death syndrome: results from 1993-5 case-control study for confidential inquiry into stillbirths and death in infancy', *BMJ*, vol 313, pp 195-9.

Bonellie, S.R. (2001) 'Effect of maternal age, smoking and deprivation on birthweight', *Paediatric and Perinatal Epidemiology*, vol 15, pp 19-26.

Brunner, E. (1997) 'Stress and the biology of inequality', *BMJ*, vol 314, pp 1472-6.

Davey Smith, G., Bartley, M. and Blane, D. (1990a) 'The Black Report on socio-economic inequalities in health 10 years on', *BMJ*, vol 301, pp 373-7.

Davey Smith, G., Morris, J.N. and Shaw, M. (1998) 'The independent inquiry into inequalities in health: a worthy successor to the Black Report?', *BMJ*, vol 317, pp 1465-6.

Davey Smith, G., Shipley, M.J. and Rose, G. (1990b) 'Magnitude and causes of socioeconomic differentials in mortality: further evidence from the Whitehall Study', *Journal of Epidemiology and Community Health*, vol 44, no 4, pp 265-70.

DH (Department of Health) (1992) *The health of the nation: A strategy for health in England*, London: HMSO.

DH (1996) *Variations in health: What can the Department of Health and the NHS do?*, London: DH.

DH (2003) *Tackling health inequalities: A Programme for Action*, London: The Stationery Office.

DH (2004) *Choosing health: Making healthier choices easier*, Cm 6374, London: The Stationery Office.

DH (2005) *Tackling health inequalities: Status report on the Programme for Action*, London: DH (www.dh.gov.uk, accessed 6 March 2006).

Dowler, E. and Calvert, C. (1995) *Nutrition and diet in lone-parent families*, London: Family Policy Studies Centre.

Dyer, O. (2005) 'Disparities in health widen between rich and poor in England', *BMJ*, vol 331, p 419.

Exworthy, M., Stuart, M., Blane, D. and Marmot, M. (2003) *Tackling health inequalities since the Acheson Inquiry*, Bristol: The Policy Press.

Forsdahl, A. (1977) 'Are poor living conditions in childhood and adolescent an important risk factor for arteriosclerotic heart disease?', *British Journal of Preventive and Social Medicine*, vol 31, no 2, pp 91-5.

Graham, H. (1994) 'Gender and class as dimensions of smoking behaviour in Britain: insights from a survey of mothers', *Social Science and Medicine*, vol 38, no 5, pp 691-8.

Harding, S. and Balarajan, R. (2000) 'Limiting long-term illness among black Caribbeans, black Africans, Indians, Pakistanis, Bangladeshis, and Chinese born in the UK', *Ethnic Health*, vol 5, no 1, pp 41-6.

Hogan, D.P., Msall, M.E., Rogers, M.L. and Avery, R.C. (1997) 'Improved disability population estimates of functional limitation among American children aged 5-17', *Maternal and Child Health*, vol 1, no 4, pp 203-6.

Hunter, D.J. (2005) 'Choosing or losing health?', *Journal of Epidemiology and Community Health*, vol 59, no 12, pp 1010-13.

Ineichen, B. (1993) *Homes and health: How housing and health interact*, London: E&FN Spon.

Jenkins, S.P. and Rigg, J.A. (2003) *Disability and disadvantage: Selection, onset and duration effects*, CASEpaper 74, London: Centre for Analysis of Social Exclusion, London School of Economics.

Kawachi, I., Kennedy, B.P., Lochner, K. and Prothrow-Smith, D. (1997) 'Social capital, income inequality and mortality', *American Journal of Public Health*, vol 87, no 9, pp 1491-8.

Kennedy, B.P., Kawachi, I. and Prothrow-Smith, D. (1996) 'Income distribution and mortality: cross sectional ecological study of the Robin Hood index in the United States', *BMJ*, vol 312, pp 1004-7.

Kuh, D. and Ben-Shlomo, Y. (eds) (1997) *A life course approach to chronic disease epidemiology*, Oxford: Oxford University Press.

Lobstein, T. (1997) *Myths about food and low income*, London: National Food Alliance (www.sustainweb.org/publications/downloads/pov_myths.pdf, accessed 4 March 2006).

Lowry, S. (1991) *Housing and health*, London: BMJ Publications.

Lynch, J.W., Davey Smith, G., Kaplan, G.A. and House, J.S. (2000) 'Income inequality and mortality: importance to health of individual income, psychosocial environment and material conditions', *BMJ*, vol 320, pp 1200-4.

Marmot, M. (2004) *Status syndrome*, London: Bloomsbury.

Marmot, M., Bosma, H., Hemingway, H., Brunner, E. and Stansfeld, S. (1997) 'Contribution of job control and other risk factors to social variations in coronary heart disease incidence', *Lancet*, vol 350, no 9073, pp 235-9.

McLoone, P. and Boddy, F.A. (1994) 'Deprivation and mortality in Scotland, 1981 to 1991', *BMJ*, vol 309, pp 1465-70.

Nazroo, J. (2003) 'The structuring of ethnic inequalities in health: economic position, racial discrimination, and racism', *American Journal of Public Health*, vol 93, no 2, pp 277-84.

NCH (National Children's Homes) (1991) *Poverty and nutrition survey 1991*, London: NCH Action for Children.

Paneth, N. (1995) 'The problems of low birth weight', *The Future of Children*, vol 5, no 1, pp 20-32.

Power, C. and Matthews, S. (1997) 'Origins of health inequalities in a national population sample', *Lancet*, vol 350, pp 1584-9.

Power, C., Manor, O. and Fox, J. (1991) *Health and class: The early years*, London: Chapman & Hall.

Sameroff, A.J. and Suomi, S.J. (1996) 'Primates and persons: a comparative developmental understanding of social organization', in R.B. Cairns, G.H. Elder and E.J. Costello (eds) *Developmental Science*, Cambridge: Cambridge University Press, pp 97-120.

Shaw, M., Dorling, D., Gordon, D. and Davey Smith, G. (1999) *The widening gap: Health inequalities and policy in Britain*, Bristol: The Policy Press.

Shaw, M., Dorling, D., Mitchell, R. and Davey Smith, G. (2005) 'Labour's "Black report" moment?', *BMJ*, vol 331, p 575.

Spencer, N.J. (2003) *Weighing the evidence: How is birthweight determined?* Oxford: Radcliffe Press.

Spencer, N.J., Bambang, S., Logan, S. and Gill, L. (1999a) 'Socioeconomic status and birth weight: comparison of an area-based measure with the Registrar General's social class', *Journal of Epidemiology and Community Health*, vol 53, pp 495-8.

Spencer, N.J., Logan, S., and Gill, L. (1999b) 'Trends and social patterning of birthweight in Sheffield, 1985-94', *Archives of Disease in Childhood*, vol 81, pp F138-F140.

Strand, B.H. and Tverdal, A. (2004) 'Can cardiovascular risk factors and lifestyle explain the educational inequalities in mortality from ischaemic heart disease and from other heart diseases? 26 year follow up of 50,000 Norwegian men and women', *Journal of Epidemiology and Community Health*, vol 58, no 8, pp 705-9.

Townsend, P and Davidson, N. (1982) *Inequalities in health: The Black Report*, Harmondsworth: Penguin.

Wanless, D. (2002) *Securing our future health: Taking a long-term view. Final report*, London: HM Treasury (www.hm-treasury.gov.uk/consultations_and_legislation/wanless/consult_wanless_final.cfm).

Wanless, D. (2004) *Securing good health for the whole population. Final report*, London: HMSO (www.hm-treasury.gov.uk/consultations_and_legislation/wanless/consult_wanless04_final.cfm).

Wilkinson, R. (1996) *Unhealthy societies: The afflictions of inequality*, London: Routledge.

Williams, D.R. (1992) 'Black-White differences in blood pressure: the role of social factors', *Ethnicity and Disease*, vol 2, no 2, pp 126-41.

# TWO

# Progress in tackling health inequalities: a policy maker's reflections

*Ray Earwicker*

Health inequalities were identified in 1997 as a priority for the new government elected in May of that year. Prime Minister Tony Blair told the House of Commons that 'inequalities do matter and there is no doubt that the published statistics show a link between income, inequality and poor health. It is important to address that issue and we are doing so' (*Hansard*, 1997).

This message was taken up in the home countries of the UK – in Scotland, Wales and Northern Ireland. In England, Sir Donald Acheson was commissioned to survey the position on health inequalities and identify possible responses. The result was the Acheson Report, published in November 1998 (Acheson, 1998). It has provided a cornerstone to policy development on health inequalities ever since and guided thinking in England, the rest of the UK and beyond. This chapter[1] seeks to explore how government policy has developed on health inequalities and how the Acheson Report and its recommendations have contributed to its development.

## Background

Tessa Jowell, the new Minister for Public Health, appointed to attack the root causes of ill health (Labour Party, 1997), wrote to Sir Donald Acheson, a former Chief Medical Officer for England, on 10 July. She invited him to undertake a review of health inequalities that would contribute to a new strategy for health. Sir Donald agreed to conduct the inquiry with the support of a small scientific advisory group consisting of Professor Sir Michael Marmot, Professor David Barker, Professor Hilary Graham, Professor Margaret Whitehead and Dr Jacky Chambers.

In the eyes of many, setting up the Acheson Inquiry was intended to help make good the fate of the earlier Black Report on health inequalities (DHSS, 1980). Commissioned by the last Labour government in 1977, Sir Douglas Black, a former president of the Royal College of Physicians, produced a detailed and costed blueprint for action on health inequalities. Reporting in 1980, the opportunity for translating his recommendations into action had passed, ended by a change of government in 1979.

Its recommendations were effectively buried by a limited edition release of the report on August Bank Holiday Monday (DHSS, 1980). The treatment of the report still rankled. Black remained an inspiration for those who wanted to see action on health inequalities – including many of the new Labour ministers and MPs elected in 1997.

## The Acheson Inquiry

The government welcomed the publication of the Acheson Report. Its 39 recommendations provided an agenda to reduce health inequalities. Its recommendations were interrelated, mutually supportive and the report recommended that they should be 'implemented ... on a broad front' (Acheson, 1998).

The first task of the inquiry had been to take a view about what was happening to health inequalities over recent years. Drawing on evidence from the Office for National Statistics, the report emphasised that over the past 20 years mortality between the top and bottom of the social scale had widened. 'For example, in the early 1970s, the mortality rate among men of working age was almost twice as high for those in class V (unskilled) as for those in class I (professional). By the early 1990s, it was almost three times higher' (Acheson, 1998, p 11).

The inquiry team examined next the available evidence about the causes of these inequalities and what action was effective – or likely to be effective – in narrowing the gap.

Experts were commissioned to produce papers and invited to address the inquiry, where their papers were discussed and they were cross-examined about their proposals. These 17 expert sessions covered health, social, economic and environmental issues, as well as the life course, and perspectives on ethnicity, age and gender (Gordon et al, 1999). Evidence was also received from a range of groups and individuals.

In the eyes of the inquiry team, the report's recommendations offered opportunities over time to improve the health of the less well off by action across the whole of government. It regarded three areas as crucial:

- all policies likely to have an impact on health should be evaluated in terms of their impact on health inequalities;
- a high priority should be given to the health of families with children;
- further steps should be taken to reduce income inequalities and improve the living standards of poor households (Acheson, 1998, p xi).

## Reactions to the report – two omissions

The Acheson Report received a generally favourable reception. Criticism focused on two main aspects. It was compared unfavourably against the Black Report, primarily because it failed to cost its recommendations and so provide the government with a blueprint for action.

The criticism of a lack of costed recommendations raises two points – one practical, the other political. In practical terms, it would have been difficult for a relatively short inquiry to provide detailed and credible costings for its action. Even if they could have been produced, it is likely that the debate on costings would have overshadowed any considerations of policy about what should, or could, be done. Neither did the scientific advisory group include an economist. This was not a matter of chance but the result of discussions with the minister – these discussions emphasised the need for both speed and focus. It was agreed that a scientific inquiry designed to illuminate policy options required scientists and not economists.

At the time of publication, this omission seemed like a serious political flaw. In retrospect, it is clear that the influence of the report on policy was much stronger precisely because this information was not included in the first place. A blueprint with costs attached – like the Black Report – was simply not wanted. Ministers had made this clear in the terms of reference of the inquiry that had said that the review was to be conducted 'within the overall framework of the Government's overall financial strategy' (Acheson, 1998, p 155).

In the first years of the new government, this strategy was tight. A health inequalities report, however well argued, that focused on the costs involved in the scale of action envisaged by Acheson would have been most unwelcome. Most probably, such a report would have been politely but coolly received – an important opportunity for tackling health inequalities lost, or seriously set back.

The second omission was the lack of targets. Acheson did not propose any targets, either national or local. While the potential of targets was recognised by the inquiry team, such considerations were explicitly excluded from its terms of reference. The report refers directly to this point:

> Other areas of work were omitted because they were not included in our terms of reference. So, although we recognise that the setting of targets concerned with reducing health inequalities is an important area for policy development, we were advised that consideration of this issue was not within the Inquiry's remit. (Acheson, 1998, p 3)

Targets are challenging tools for policy makers. Framing the target to produce a desirable result without undue effect elsewhere is problematic. Implementation in the real world can be even more challenging, particularly where one administrative system is replaced by another, for example where the 'command and control' system of the NHS has given way in recent years to a more devolved approach. It is even harder where action across systems or government departments is involved.

The notion of action on a 'broad front' is also complicated by departmental accountability arrangements across government departments. Each department is responsible for activities within their remit and funded by Treasury for this purpose. Cross-government action raises tricky issues. Thus, while ministers wanted to encourage a joined-up approach to government business, they were keen to avoid being pre-empted into controversy on what constituted a sensible approach to joint working without due consideration.

Both on matters of spending and targets, government caution was, at length, replaced by significant commitments in both areas.

### *Saving lives* and beyond

The Acheson Report had been commissioned to feed the forthcoming health strategy White Paper. *Saving lives: Our healthier nation* was published in 1999 and, like the Acheson Report, recognised that action to save lives, promote healthier living and reduce health inequalities required action across government (DH, 1999).

*Saving lives* provided a substantial public health agenda with a commitment to reducing health inequalities. Its starting point was to improve the health of everyone and the health of the worst off in particular. It advocated a new partnership between people, communities and government that has been a hallmark of government action in this area ever since.

The Acheson Report had served its purpose in contributing to this new health strategy. The detailed analysis in the report and the scope of its recommendations meant that it was unlikely to be relegated to a dusty shelf. Its enduring influence is a reflection of the step change in health policy brought about by the arrival of Alan Milburn as Secretary of State for Health and a loosening of the purse strings that brought new confidence to addressing NHS and wider health issues. This confidence was reflected in the decision to develop a 10-year plan for the NHS to modernise and reform the service and accommodate a wider view of health.

A new way of policy making was adopted to help meet this challenge. This plan was the product of a process that brought together academics and other experts, front-line practitioners and health service managers to work alongside senior officials and ministers in generating the ideas that underpinned it. Five groups were set up to inform this process – modernisation action teams (MATs) – with each MAT led by a minister. This approach to policy making was to have a lasting impact on the approach to tackling health inequalities that is supported by expert and lay reference groups.

## Towards a national target

The prevention and inequalities MAT was concerned with work on health inequalities. Led by Yvette Cooper, the Minister for Public Health, it considered a range of issues through a series of presentations. The MAT team was encouraged to think freely and was not burdened with terms of reference. The MAT presentations were designed to act as a spur to discussion and emergence of ideas. They were designed to absorb the lessons from practitioners about what was needed and what worked, and from experts about the evidence and the systems.

The first recommendation of the prevention and inequalities MAT was for national health inequalities targets. It argued that a plan without targets would change little – and it focused its recommendations on this proposal. A target would stake a claim for health inequalities and wider health issues and bring it to the attention of a wider audience in the NHS and beyond. In this view, the MAT was encouraged by the Acheson Report. The report had showed what could be done by government action on a broad front – only some of the levers to prompt action were missing. A national target seemed to be the logical conclusion to what Acheson was saying.

Despite the tension between the MAT proposal and established principles of accountability, *The NHS Plan* was published in July 2000. It announced that:

> For the first time ever, local targets will now be reinforced by the creation of national health inequalities targets, to narrow the gap in childhood and throughout life between socio-economic groups and between the most deprived areas and the rest of the country. Specific targets will be developed in consultation with external stakeholders and expert advice. (DH, 2000, p 106)

Several factors contributed to this decision to include health inequalities targets. There was the ambition and vision of *The NHS Plan*, the balance it struck between prevention and cure, and the strength of the MAT recommendation. Notwithstanding these factors, it still took a leap of courage from ministers to assume accountability for action outside the traditional orbit of the department for which they – and their successors – would be held accountable.

The two national health inequalities targets were announced in February 2001. They were:

> … starting with children under one year, by 2010 to reduce by at least 10 per cent the gap in mortality between manual groups and the population as a whole [and] starting with health authorities, by 2010 to reduce by at least 10 per cent the gap between the fifth of areas with the lowest life expectancy at birth and the population as a whole. (DH, 2001a)

The two elements were subsequently consolidated into a single target following the 2002 Spending Review, 'by 2010 to reduce inequalities in health outcomes by 10 per cent as measured by infant mortality and life expectancy at birth' (DH, 2003, p 7).

## A national strategy emerges

This decision on national targets was crucial in consolidating health inequalities as a priority across government, within the NHS, and with health and other professionals.

With the targets set, the next stage was to engage anyone with responsibility for, or an interest in, tackling health inequalities in a national consultation to help deliver the target. Yvette Cooper launched the consultation exercise at the King's Fund in August 2001 (DH, 2001b).

Action to meet the targets and to achieve a long-term sustainable reduction in health inequalities required cross-government engagement and, in particular, Treasury support. New three-year spending planning cycles had been introduced to encourage a more strategic approach to public spending, with Public Service Agreement (PSA) targets set to determine the results to be delivered in exchange for spending. While most discussions were conducted with departments, the health inequalities targets required a different approach and they were identified for a cross-cutting review for the 2002 Spending Review exercise. These cross-cutting reviews were set up to consider the implications of targets that required action beyond the remit of one department.

This decision had important consequences. It underlined the importance of health inequalities across government by flagging Treasury interest, providing the leadership necessary to bring the relevant government departments to the table – much more difficult for a single Whitehall department – and to build the links between them that were to underpin the future national health inequalities strategy.

Eighteen government departments and policy units were represented on this cross-cutting review. It was charged with developing the evidence base and a high-level strategy for delivery. The work of the Acheson Inquiry gave the review a head start. The summary report of the review – published in November 2002 – acknowledged that it had provided a 'firm foundation of evidence ... about the nature and scale of health inequalities' (HM Treasury and DH, 2002, p v).

This review – together with the consultation exercise – underlined the importance of assessing relevant and available evidence. Acheson provided an authoritative and useful shortcut.

The review set out a framework for a national strategy based on an approach that introduced – or mainstreamed – health inequalities into the corner of all relevant policy areas. The importance of strong government leadership, effective coordination and partnerships that looked beyond the NHS were spelt out by Hazel Blears, the new Minister for Public Health, as key themes from the consultation exercise (HM Treasury and DH, 2002, p v).

## The national strategy

Both the review and the consultation significantly shaped the national health inequalities strategy published the following year as *Tackling health inequalities: A Programme for Action* (DH, 2003). This set out plans to tackle health inequalities over the next three years, and established the foundations required to meet the target by reducing the gap in infant mortality across social groups, and raising the life expectancy in the most disadvantaged groups faster than elsewhere. It was an ambitious strategy. It declared that 'health inequalities are stubborn, persistent and difficult to change. They are also widening and will continue to do so unless we do things differently. This means addressing not only the short-term consequences of avoidable ill health but also the long term causes' (DH, 2003, p 3).

The Programme for Action was not a White Paper but it was supported by 12 government departments. In practical terms, it included 76 cross-government commitments to be delivered by 2006. They were organised across the four themes of the strategy: supporting families, mothers and children; engaging communities and individuals; preventing illness and providing effective treatment and care; and addressing the underlying determinants of health.

The Programme for Action was the culmination of a process that had started with the commissioning of the Acheson Inquiry. It brought together many of the principles that shaped Acheson – and was the fullest official expression of them. This included:

- asserting the role of the wider determinants of health – 'upstream' and well as 'downstream' factors – with its corollary of action across all levels of government;
- framing action in terms that reflected the social gradient of health rather than focusing on socially excluded groups; and,
- underlining the importance of action over the long term if policies were to achieve results.

This debt to Acheson was acknowledged in the strategy. It recognised that the inquiry had been commissioned to:

> ... understand better the causes of health inequalities, and how to tackle them ... and it has highlighted ways in which the policies and programmes of a range of government departments could have an influence on reducing health inequalities, and the potential of a more co-ordinated

approach to achieve greater synergy and impact. (DH, 2003, p 9)

The first challenge for the national strategy was to stop health inequalities from further widening. In terms of narrowing the gap, it said that 'to reduce health inequalities and achieve the targets will require us to improve the health of the poorest 30-40 per cent of the population where the greatest burden of disease exists' (DH, 2003, p 4).

The national strategy meant a new focus. It no longer emphasised targeting aimed at specific and needy groups, though this still might be required in some circumstances. Instead, the main thrust would be for a strategic approach that looked at health inequalities issues in the round by mainstreaming action through the whole range of public and other services. This was challenging, requiring changes of perception and practice among policy makers and practitioners, but unless this happened health inequalities would continue to widen.

To help achieve this shift, the Programme for Action stressed the need to assign roles and responsibilities for action across the four themes, and assess and monitor the impact of activity through public service performance management systems, particularly in the NHS.

It was clear that results would take time, but the Prime Minister made clear the government's commitment 'to deliver long-term improvement, through investment, reform and local responsibility, in the health and health care of the most disadvantaged in our society' (DH, 2003, p 1).

Time lags in data can obscure the early results of effective action in the short term. But the Programme for Action also stressed the inter-generational aspects of many of the factors contributing to health inequalities that would require many years to change. This underlaid the twin-track approach that was at the heart of the strategy, namely to help meet the 2010 target and achieve a long-term sustainable reduction in health inequalities.

## Building on the strategy

The strategy marked a watershed between understanding the causes of health inequalities and doing something about them. This meant addressing the systems and processes that would facilitate change. The consequence was a greater emphasis on the levers to promote action and partnership at local, regional and central government level – and a greater emphasis on the 2010 target. At the same time, there was growing recognition that action on tackling health inequalities was necessary if best value was to be achieved from increased health spending. This increased the urgency for taking a wider view of health.

Derek Wanless, a former chief executive of National Westminster Bank, was commissioned by the Treasury to consider these issues (HM Treasury, 2004). He argued that only a population that was 'fully engaged' in improving its health would ensure best value from health spending. The government would be unable to meet its public health goals – and incur considerable extra and avoidable NHS expenditure – if it failed to provide more, and more effective, help to the most deprived groups in society. The report said that:

> The burden of disease is disproportionately borne by these groups because of the social gradient in risk factors like smoking and obesity, which contribute to a higher incidence of diseases like cancer, diabetes and heart disease. In order to tackle this concern and maximise the impact of interventions, a focus on health inequalities will be key to the government's public health approach. (HM Treasury, 2004, p 95)

In response to this concern, the 2004 Spending Review added a health inequalities dimension to the PSA targets for heart disease, stroke and related diseases, and for cancer. This required the incidence of these diseases to be narrowed between the fifth of areas with the worst health and deprivation indicators and the population as a whole, mirroring the life expectancy element of the health inequalities target. Monitoring planning and performance would be crucial to effective local action. In July 2004, a new NHS planning and performance framework, *National standards, local action* (DH, 2004a), announced a major change in the way the NHS would address health issues. John Reid, the new Secretary of State for Health, made it clear that the 'focus of NHS reform is now shifting to improving the quality of care patients receive. The NHS will develop into a health service rather than one that focuses primarily on sickness. There will be a sustained drive to reduce inequalities in health. There will be few national targets and greater scope for local organisations to tackle local priorities' (DH, 2004a, p 3).

Specifically, this meant designing local targets that delivered equity. A new public health standard was set in the guidance that called on healthcare organisations to identify health inequality issues and implement effective programmes to improve and reduce health inequalities, a standard that would be assessed by the Healthcare Commission.

A strong sense of momentum had been developed in the months following the publication of the national strategy. Against a background of an array of health policy initiatives, it can be difficult to strike a balance between messages for improving the health of the population and those for tackling health inequalities. Acheson had noted that too strong an emphasis on general health improvement can widen the health gap (Acheson, 1998, p 30). The White Paper *Choosing health: Making healthy choices easier* (DH, 2004b) exemplified this difficulty. Published in November 2004, it was founded on the twin pillars of health improvement and health inequalities. The emphasis on personal health and choice, however, was seen as stressing health improvement at the expense of health inequalities. The health inequalities messages in *Choosing health* were there but not always received (DH, 2004b, p 106). A stronger emphasis on health inequalities in the White Paper would, however, have helped sustain momentum and deflect any misleading impression that health inequalities were marginal to the wider public health agenda.

*Delivering 'Choosing health'*, the plan for delivering the White Paper commitments, helped rectify any such impression by listing health inequalities first on its list of priorities (DH, 2005a). More recently, health inequalities have been identified as a top six NHS priority. This will provide a stronger alignment between the health inequalities and health improvement agendas, and recognition of the role of health inequalities in the NHS (see Chapters Three, Four and Five for contrasting views of *Choosing health* and its underlying philosophy).

## Future action

The elevation of health inequalities to the position of a top six NHS priority means that there should be a much stronger NHS focus on the issue. Sitting alongside some of the most important acute sector priorities, it enhances the prospect of stopping the health inequalities gap widening further and meeting the 2010 target, not least when it is combined with action in the most disadvantaged parts of the country through the spearhead group of the 70 local authority areas – covering 28% of the population – with the worst health and deprivation indicators, and the health inequalities dimension of local area agreements being adopted by local authorities.

It is clear, however, that progress will not be easy. The *Status report on the Programme for Action*, published in August 2005 (DH, 2005b), provided a first review of data against the 2010 PSA target, the 12 national headline indicators and the set of departmental commitments included in the strategy. Covering developments up to 2003, it showed no narrowing of health inequalities against the PSA target. There was a continuing widening of these inequalities as measured by infant mortality and life expectancy reflecting the long-term trend; however, there were:

> ... signs that some of the indicators associated with health inequalities are moving in the right direction. The progress achieved in tackling and significantly reducing child poverty will contribute to health inequalities in the future. It shows how a well designed, focused and strongly supported programme can achieve change over time. (DH, 2005b, p 1)

The status report gave a view of the position as at the date of the publication of the strategy. Caroline Flint, the Minister for Public Health, stressed that there 'is no room for complacency. Reversing the trend in inequalities will need a sustained commitment at national and local level. This report shows how far we have to go, and it helps signal the way' (DH, 2005b, p 2).

## Conclusion

This chapter has considered how government action on health inequalities has developed in England since 1997, and how the Acheson Report helped shape these developments. Looking back from the perspective of the UK presidency of the EU in the second half of 2005, it was seen that the 'publication of the Acheson report in 1998 ... marked a new surge of interest in health inequalities in England and elsewhere' (Mackenbach, 2006, p 5).

Acheson laid the foundation for what followed – the targets and the national strategy. The style and content of the report has meant that it is still influential. The reasons for this are as follows: first, the explicitly independent and scientific nature of the report – it cites over 600 scientific sources to underpin its arguments; second, its broad view of influences on health inequalities – and the need for a response 'on a broad front' if health inequalities are to be reduced on a long-term and sustainable basis; third, its focus, which went beyond the socially excluded to encompass a much larger part of the population and recognised that health inequalities affect many working families; and fourth, its authoritative nature, which has provided the opportunity to shift the debate from analysing the causes of health inequalities to prescriptions for tackling them. Acheson illustrated the point that while it is important to understand the nature of the world, it is also important to use that knowledge to change it. The report's expert – non-political – nature has also contributed to its continuing influence.

Developing a national strategy with support across government has been a significant achievement. A new set of challenges faces the strategy over the next few years. An accelerated effort will be needed to maintain the momentum to meet the 2010 target. Sustaining the wider agenda for social justice, continuing to secure a reduction in poverty – including child poverty – and improvements in housing, employment and education, will be the bedrock on which this effort will be built. The role of the NHS is crucial and the top six status of health inequalities is a sign that this has been recognised.

A closer focus will also be needed on the local mechanics of change. This means doing things differently, for example seeking out and sharing good practice that will help narrow the gap across a range of interventions shown to contribute to narrowing the gap, and delivering them on an appropriate scale. It also means building effective local partnerships that engage the NHS, local government and other key players. The closer match between the NHS and local government areas arising from the NHS reconfiguration will help facilitate these opportunities. Moving towards the target will be important because it will show that evidence-based action that is targeted and delivered appropriately can have an impact on health inequalities, narrow the gap and improve the lives of disadvantaged people in a way that encourages ministers across government and others to persevere with the fight towards a long-term sustainable reduction in health inequalities.

## Note
[1] The author works in the Health Inequalities Unit at the Department of Health and was secretary to the Acheson Inquiry on inequalities in health (1997-98). However, he is writing here in a personal capacity and his views in no way represent those of the department.

## References

Acheson, D. (1998) *Independent inquiry into inequalities in health*, London: The Stationery Office.

DH (Department of Health) (1999) *Saving lives: Our healthier nation*, Cm 4386, London: The Stationery Office.

DH (2000) *The NHS Plan: A plan for investment, a plan for reform*, London: The Stationery Office.

DH (2001a) 'Health Secretary announces new plans to improve health in the poorest areas', DH press release, 1 August.

DH (2001b) *Tackling health inequalities: Consultation on a plan for delivery*, London: DH.

DH (2002) *Tackling health inequalities: The results of the consultation exercise*, London: DH.

DH (2003) *Tackling health inequalities: A Programme for Action*, London: DH.

DH (2004a) *National standards, local action*, London: DH.

DH (2004b) *Choosing health: Making healthier choices easier*, Cm 6374, London: The Stationery Office.

DH (2005a) *Delivering 'Choosing health'*, London: DH.

DH (2005b) *Tackling health inequalities: Status report on the Programme for Action*, London: DH.

DHSS (Department of Health and Social Security) (1980) *Inequalities in health: Report of a research working group* (Black Report), London: DHSS.

Gordon, D. et al (1999) *Inequalities in health: Evidence presented to the independent inquiry into inequalities in health*, Bristol: The Policy Press.

*Hansard* (1997) House of Commons, 11 June, cols 1139-40.

HM Treasury (2004) *2004 Spending Review*, London: The Stationery Office.

HM Treasury and DH (2002) *Tackling health inequalities: Summary of the 2002 cross-cutting review*, London: DH.

Labour Party (1997) *Because Britain deserves better*, new Labour Manifesto, London: The Labour Party.

Mackenbach, J. (2006) *Health inequalities: Europe in profile*, London: Department of Health.

# THREE

# Inequalities in mortality rates under New Labour

*Danny Dorling, Mary Shaw and George Davey Smith*

## Introduction: learn to talk like me and be an angel too

> Things can only get better
> they can only get better, now I found you
> Things can only get better, they can only get better,
> now I found you
> and you and you
> You have shown me prejudice and greed
> And you've shown me how I must learn to deal with this
> disease
> I look at things now in a different light than I did before
> And I've found the cause
> and I think you can be my cure
> So teach me to ...
> Walk your path, wear your shoes, talk like that, I'll be an angel
> and
> Things can only get better ...
>                     (www.lyricsdownload.com/d-ream-things-can-only-
>                                          get-better-lyrics.html)

New Labour came to power in 1997 to the theme of D:Ream's 'Things can only get better'. As the lyrics to its campaign tune said, it thought that it had found the cause of all that was wrong in Britain and that it was the party that would be the cure to the disease of prejudice and greed. It was going to be an angel – and things could only get better.

Prior to 1997, throughout the long 18 years of Conservative government, Labour had referred to the issue of increasing social inequalities in health as an area of particular concern. Thus it was surely a good sign that before the May 1997 election it had announced that it would launch an independent inquiry into inequalities in health.

The inquiry was launched in July 1997, with Tessa Jowell, the new Minister for Public Health, criticising the health strategy of the previous administration for 'its excessive emphasis on lifestyle issues', which 'cast the responsibility back on to the individual' (DH, 1997). She gave a commitment regarding the inquiry's findings that these 'conclusions, based on evidence, will contribute to the development of a new strategy for health' (DH, 1997).

The independent inquiry report duly appeared (Acheson, 1998). It presented a wealth of evidence on the extent and trends of inequalities in health. This, together with a large body of other evidence drawn together in the report, demonstrated clearly that the previous two decades had seen large and growing inequalities in income in Britain, and that these had been accompanied by equally stark increases in health inequalities and in life chances more generally defined. The main task of the inquiry had been to produce recommendations for policies that could alleviate inequalities in health. Some 39 recommendations, many with sets of sub-recommendations, were given. While they contain some focused policies, the overall force of the recommendations was considerably weakened by a lack of prioritisation; by being inadequately concrete; and by being uncosted (Davey Smith et al, 1998).

Because the recommendations were not presented in any hierarchy, the essential fact that inequalities in health followed closely on inequalities in wealth was under-emphasised. In fact, inequalities in wealth continued to rise under New Labour well into its third term and will almost certainly continue to increase beyond that (Dorling et al, 2005). The recommendations on the necessity to 'reduce poverty and income inequalities' thus appeared at the time to have similar status to those concerned with reducing traffic speed, or offering concessionary fares to pensioners. The fundamental role of inequalities in material circumstances producing inequalities in other exposures and outcomes was therefore missed, and it became a possibility that many of the report's recommendations could be adopted – at least nominally – without addressing the underlying determinants of health inequalities.

Many of the sets of recommendations were also too vague to be useful. Recommending 'measures to prevent suicide among young people, especially among young men and seriously mentally ill people', or 'the development of policies to reduce the fear of crime and violence, and to create a safe environment for people to live in' received universal support, but they were of little use in practice since it was not specified how these things were to be brought about. Rates of violence in Britain subsequently rose under New Labour, although suicide rates did not

(Hillyard et al, 2005). As an example of how the recommendations were inadequately concrete, the report advocates the development of a high-quality public transport system that is affordable to the user and specifically refers to the large relative increases in rail fares compared with motoring costs, but it failed to make the obvious link with the privatisation of the railways. Rail prices have subsequently risen, as the railways were not renationalised (Dorling, 2005, p xv).

Lastly, as the recommendations were not costed, it was impossible to evaluate the relative costs of their implementation, the predicted social benefits that would follow and the opportunity costs of not investing in other areas. This lack of costing allowed the key recommendations to be side-stepped by implying that they were unrealistic and could not be implemented in the current economic climate (Davey Smith et al, 1998).

The previous major report on inequalities in health had been that of the committee chaired by Sir Douglas Black (which produced the so-called Black Report (DHSS, 1980)), commissioned by the previous Labour government in 1977 and reporting to the then new Conservative administration in 1980. The Black Report discussed the inequalities in health and in income that existed at the time and made a series of policy recommendations. These were rejected by Patrick Jenkin, then Secretary of State for Social Services, as being unrealistic; the report was deliberately released before a national holiday, with no press release or press conference, and with only 260 copies produced. (It was subsequently published as a paperback (Townsend and Davidson, 1982) and widely read.)

For 17 of the 18 years of Conservative government, the Labour Party had made political capital out of the non-implementation of the recommendations of the Black Report. The report's enthusiasm for addressing inequalities in health appeared to be one element that survived the transformation from Old to New Labour. A few weeks before the May 1997 Labour election victory, Baroness Jay had stated that the Black Report 'provided the essential base and policy guide to any responsible government wanting to take action' on inequalities in health (*Hansard*, 1997). She then committed the incoming Labour government to a health strategy in which the distribution of economic resources would be a key element (DHSS, 1980). In the same debate, another Labour peer had stated that the 'failure since 1980 to implement any of the Black Report recommendations has caused disappointment to many and must have caused a great deal of needless suffering on the part of many of the poorest families' (Hansard, 1997).

Thus, following the election landslide of 1997 and in the light of

Labour's long-term declared policy on inequalities in health, it was very disappointing that a major limitation on the Acheson Inquiry was its brief from the government, which stated that it had to be carried out 'within the broad framework of the Government's overall financial strategy' (see preamble to Acheson, 1998). This set the stage for what happened next and constrained the inquiry from proposing markedly redistributive fiscal policies, given the commitments on taxation made by Labour prior to the 1997 election.

In understanding the position New Labour inherited, it is worth remembering that the Black Report was commissioned in 1977, when inequalities in income were in fact at an historic low point. In 1977, only 7% of the population were on incomes below half of the average after housing costs; by 1995/96 this had more than trebled to 24% (DSS, 1998) (where it remains, give or take a percentage point, today). The increasing inequalities in income – which saw the UK lead the developed world in income inequality and child poverty (Lynch and Kaplan, 1997) – started under the last Labour government, in 1977. Twenty years later, Tony Blair declared that 'I believe in greater equality. If the Labour government has not raised the living standards of the poorest by the end of its time in office it will have failed' (Howarth et al, 1998). However, the New Labour strategy of saying one thing and doing another was already clear. When the report of the inquiry was commissioned, it was done with the constraint that its recommendations needed to fall within the broad framework of the government's overall financial strategy (Black et al, 1999; Davey Smith et al, 1999). Since this strategy included maintaining the overall fiscal plans of the previous Conservative administration, this meant no increase in taxation and therefore excluded the major strategy to reduce inequalities in income. After nearly two decades of the Labour Party out of office promoting the implementation of the recommendations of the Black Report, the commissioning of a new report with such constraints applied in advance was in fact a step backwards, although, with characteristic New Labour spin, the commissioning was presented as demonstrating commitment to the cause of reducing inequalities, rather than as the first of a number of side-steps of the central issue of inequality in income and wealth.

## Midterm: we'll get up and start again

> Lifted up today, lifted all the way, yeah we could be lifted
> We could be lifted from the shadows, we could be lifted
> Lifted up to new horizons
> When it all gets dark again, it doesn't really matter 'bout the
> rain
> When it all gets dark again, it doesn't really matter 'bout the
> rain
>
> (www.lyricsdepot.com/lighthouse-family/lifted.html)

New Labour went on to win the 2001 general election, its theme tune courtesy of The Lighthouse Family. Although its policies relating to social inequality had been criticised, too little time had passed since 1997, it was argued, for their actual effect to be monitored (Dorling, 2006). There was also no serious political alternative to Labour, and its reputation and record did not yet appear tarnished (even if it had chosen a campaign song with the chorus 'We could be lifted' and ending '... when it all gets dark again, it doesn't really matter 'bout the rain'). The widening gap between rich and poor continued to grow.

The widening gap in health by social class could be seen not only in the mortality rates of adults, but also in that of infants (see Chapter Five for a further discussion of the trends in infant and child health inequalities). In fact, it was the infant mortality rate that Labour expected to improve most quickly as that was not in any straightforward way affected by, for instance, the lagged impact of smoking rates 20 years earlier. In his last report as Chief Medical Officer on the state of the public health, Sir Kenneth Calman in 1997 highlighted in his introduction a number of overall improvements in health, including the fact that infant mortality had fallen to its lowest recorded rate of 5.9 deaths per 1,000 live births (DH, 1998). However, a closer inspection of these rates revealed that, while overall infant mortality rates had levelled off in the four years prior to 1997, when these rates were considered by social class (of father), a different picture emerged. As Figure 3.1a shows, there were growing differences between the death rates of babies with social class I fathers (professional occupations) and babies with social class V fathers (unskilled manual workers) – babies of unskilled manual workers were 2.2 times more likely to die than babies with fathers in professional occupations. For every 1,000 babies born whose father was social class V, eight babies died within their first year.

These trends were based on only a few years of data when they were first reported (Davey Smith et al, 1999) – because of changes in how data are reported – and a relatively small number (statistically speaking) of deaths. Therefore, it was important to monitor the infant mortality rate by social class over the coming years to see if this trend continued. In fact, this infant mortality indicator was used as a government target, and as Figure 3.1b shows, the excess mortality rate of the more widely defined infants in the 'routine and manual' class actually fell when compared with 'all' between 1996 and 1997, and 1997 and 1998. Unfortunately, after that it rose fairly relentlessly.

Although the new infant mortality figures were not released in full until 2005, in New Labour's third term, it had become obvious during

**Figure 3.1a: Infant mortality by social class, 1993-96**

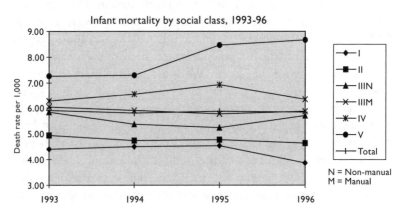
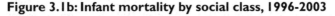

**Figure 3.1b: Infant mortality by social class, 1996-2003**

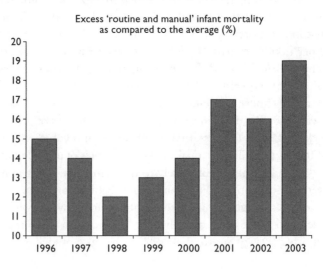

the second term that mortality inequalities were not declining between areas. In fact, as Table 3.1 shows, they had reached an all-time high by the first two years of the New Labour government, but the lag time in releasing and analysing data meant that that this was not known until its second term (Davey Smith et al, 2002).

Thus inequalities in health were rising both between social class for infants and between areas for premature mortality during both the first and second terms of the government, despite its pledge to reduce those inequalities as a priority.

Although a great deal could be written about what Labour did do in its first and second terms, that would detract from what actually happened on the ground as, despite a great many fine words, inequalities became worse. The Labour government itself has also written reams and reams of reports and papers on what it has done. We could also speculate about what might have happened had Labour not won power in 1997 and again in 2001, but it did win power. By this time, Labour had become obsessed with its image and was releasing statistics showing that everything it measured was getting better everywhere (this is not an exaggeration: see Dorling et al, 2002)). It was perhaps no coincidence that its third campaign theme song included the line 'I know I'm not a hopeless case'. It had begun to believe its own spin.

**Table 3.1: Spatial inequality in mortality in Britain, 1990-99**

| Age and sex standardised mortality ratios (SMRs) (0-74) according to decile of poverty, and the relative index of inequality (RII) | | | | | |
|---|---|---|---|---|---|
| SMR 0-74 | 1990-91 | 1992-93 | 1994-95 | 1996-97 | 1998-99 |
| Decile 1 | 129 | 132 | 134 | 136 | 138 |
| Decile 2 | 117 | 119 | 118 | 120 | 122 |
| Decile 3 | 110 | 112 | 111 | 113 | 114 |
| Decile 4 | 109 | 109 | 109 | 110 | 111 |
| Decile 5 | 101 | 100 | 100 | 101 | 103 |
| Decile 6 | 96 | 95 | 96 | 95 | 97 |
| Decile 7 | 92 | 91 | 91 | 92 | 92 |
| Decile 8 | 87 | 88 | 87 | 87 | 87 |
| Decile 9 | 85 | 83 | 84 | 84 | 83 |
| Decile 10 | 81 | 81 | 81 | 80 | 80 |
| RII | 1.68 | 1.74 | 1.75 | 1.80 | 1.85 |

*Source:* Davey Smith et al (2002).

The second term was also when the Labour government went to war, hand in hand with George Bush's US government, in Afghanistan and Iraq. It was also in this term that Tony Blair increased his own pay by 41% in one year (Grice, 2001). Inequalities in wealth continued to rise (Wintour, 2004).

## Third term: I know I'm not a hopeless case

> It was a beautiful day
> Don't let it get away
> Beautiful day
> Touch me
> Take me to that other place
> Reach me
> I know I'm not a hopeless case
> What you don't have you don't need it now
> What you don't know you can feel it somehow
> What you don't have you don't need it now
> Don't need it now
> Was a beautiful day
>             (www.seeklyrics.com/lyrics/U2/Beautiful-Day.html)

Labour chose a song from U2 as its third campaign theme to help it secure the general election of 2005. Shortly after it won that election on a depleted majority, it secured its own 'Black Report' moment. This came with the release of the government's then long-promised report on health inequalities: *Tackling health inequalities: Status report on the Programme for Action*, released on 11 August 2005 (DH, 2005a). In July 2003, the government had stated that there would be an annual report from the Department of Health's Health Inequality Unit on health inequality indicators in relation to the health inequality targets. Nothing appeared for more than two years; then, conveniently soon after the 2005 election and two years after the promise of an annual report, the status report finally appeared. The eventual release was also a curious affair. It was reminiscent of the deliberately covert release of the Black Report on an August Bank Holiday Monday in 1980, discussed earlier. The status report also appeared at a time when the responsible Minister – Caroline Flint, Minister for Public Health – was on holiday, and her deputy was unavailable. Even stranger, the press release referring to the report (DH, 2005b) deflected attention from the key finding of widening inequalities in life expectancy and infant mortality by headlining that 12 'early adopter sites' were to be the first areas to have 'health trainers'.

Caroline Flint said in the press release that: 'Many people have difficulty in changing to a healthier way of life … Health trainers are one of the many initiatives in the White Paper which will help narrow this gap by supporting people to make healthier choices in their daily lives' (DH, 2005b). To Labour Party traditionalists, opposed to victim-blaming approaches to health promotion, this must have triggered memories of Conservative minister Edwina Currie admonishing the poor to buy cheap but healthy food (Shaw et al, 2005a). To New Labour, however – by the end of the second term any admonition of greed having disappeared, relaxed about the rich getting richer (Blair, 2001) and comfortable with the wholesale adoption of Conservative ideology – it was perhaps grist to the mill.

The scientific endorsement of the report was also at odds with its key findings. After years of making seminal contributions to the study of the 'social gradient' in mortality, the chair of the Scientific Reference Group on Health Inequalities, the eminent epidemiologist Sir Michael Marmot implied that current inequalities within England were insignificant in comparison with marked historical improvements and international comparisons:

**Figure 3.2: Inequalities in life expectancy between the best- and worst-off districts of Britain, 1999-2004**

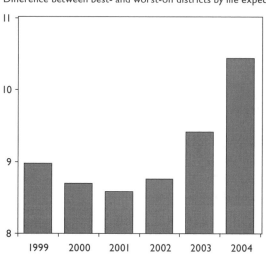

Difference between best- and worst-off districts by life expectancy (years)

*Source:* Dorling (2006)

> Now we're talking about an average of five per 1,000 live births for the country and in the worst off areas it's six. It sounds like a scandal; why hasn't it got better? But in fact we're looking at the most dramatic improvement... The worst off group is six per 1,000 live births. The best in the world is Iceland at three per 1,000 live births, the worst in the world is Sierra Leone with 196, so on a scale from Iceland to Sierra Leone the worst off in Britain is six. They're very close to the Iceland figures. (Marmot, 2005)

Of course, such comparisons do add sobering perspective to the extent of inequalities within England, but it was strange to hear the chair of the Scientific Reference Group on Health Inequalities dismiss inequalities within his own society so easily. Even the most conservative measures of inequalities in health between large areas in England show that all infants in poorer areas are at least twice as likely to die in their first year of life than those in more affluent areas (ONS, 2005). If the comparisons are made between smaller areas and between the chances of babies born to affluent couples versus those whose birth is registered to a poorer single parent or to parents in lower social classes, the inequalities are considerably more stark than the headline figure (see also Chapter Five for a discussion of the limitations of comparing infant mortality among the most disadvantaged with the average rather than the least disadvantaged). Similarly, the growing life expectancy difference between areas (Shaw et al, 2005b) equates to millions of years of life ended prematurely every year in the United Kingdom. To imply that the suffering caused as inequalities worsen is 'minimal' is surely misleading, and contrasts with Sir Michael Marmot's comments a year earlier:

> In 2004 it is not acceptable – at least to me – that life expectancy should decline by a year for each of the next six stops you travel eastwards along the London Underground District Line from Tower Hill in the East End. Talking about individual choice in health makes good political rhetoric. But the scientific reality is that peoples' choices are determined by their social arrangements and life circumstances. (Marmot, 2004, p 11)

In fact, the circumstances of the report's release fortunately did not in the end detract from its main message – that health inequalities, as measured by both spatial differences in life expectancy and socioeconomic differences in infant mortality, had widened. The latest data for life expectancy (2001-03) then available showed that the gap between England as a whole and the fifth of local authorities with the lowest life expectancy had increased, by 2% for males and by 5% for females (DH, 2005a). Inequalities continued to rise throughout 2004, as Figure 3.2 summarises. Likewise, around 1995, babies of working-class parents had been 15% more likely to die in their first year of life compared with all infants; that rate of inequality fell to a low of 12% by 1997 but rose again to its maximum of 19% by 2003, which was the latest year of data available for the report.

For the first time we also learnt from the report that, apparently, these poor results were to be expected: 'There is, as expected over this short timescale, no narrowing of health inequalities against the PSA target. There is a continued widening of these inequalities as measured by infant mortality and life expectancy, reflecting the long-term trend' (DH, 2005a, p 1). Thus, despite the publication of the Acheson Report in 1998 (Acheson, 1998), a raft of policy documents since and an historic third term for Labour, it is still *apparently* too early to expect change, as 'many interventions will only be coming on stream after 2003' (DH, 2005a, p 6). Expectations thus seem to have dwindled since the heady days of 'things can only get better', 'I believe in greater equality' (Tony Blair in 1996) (Shaw et al, 1999) and 'the whole Government, led from the top by the Prime Minister, is committed to the greatest ever reduction in health inequalities' (Frank Dobson, then Health Secretary in 1998, quoted in Shaw et al, 1999).

The assessment of trends in health inequalities was not helped by the shifting sands of the targets themselves, which had their spatial and social units altered, their start dates changed and measures adjusted repeatedly (for a contrasting view of targets, see Chapter Two). The life expectancy target first mentioned 'health authorities', which were soon abolished, then, the 'fifth of local authorities with the lowest life expectancy', and now referred to a slightly different 'spearhead' group. Curiously, the 12 'early adopter sites' that are to get 'health trainers' overlap with (but are not exclusively drawn from) the 'spearhead' group. Thus the spearhead group will (for) now be used to measure progress towards the life expectancy target. The infant mortality target has likewise been reformulated, as the official measure of social class has changed. Moreover, neither of the targets are true health inequalities targets as they compare the worst-off groups with the average for the population as a whole, rather than considering the entire distribution. Indeed, the rapid 'moving of the goalposts' seems to have confused the drafters of the status report, with 2001, 2002 and 2003 being given at various points as when the targets were set (DH, 2005a). In fact, the first New Labour health inequalities target was given in February 2001 and, even then, the wording was quite complex (DH, 2001).

As we outlined at the beginning of the chapter, in opposition Labour consistently promised to implement the recommendations of the Black Report and were incensed at the shoddy attempt made to cover it up, as they were by the similar attempt to suppress the impact of the follow-up *Health divide* in 1987 (Berridge, 2002). The fear raised by the hushed-up release of this 2005 status report was that the bold statements and unprecedented promises of New Labour's first years in power (for example, the pledge to eradicate child poverty within a generation (Waugh, 1999)) have been wholly overtaken by the individualistic rhetoric of behavioural prevention and 'choosing health', with its three principles of 'informed choice, personalisation, and working together' (DH, 2004). The linking of the adverse trends in health inequalities with the introduction of health trainers is a prime example of why this anxiety has grown (coupled with comments of the Prime Minister such as those quoted below in the conclusion to this chapter). While the proportion of children living in low-income households is a national indicator (Dorling, 2006), nowhere in the status report is there any mention of measuring, let alone directly tackling, the static or widening inequalities in income and wealth over which New Labour has presided – with widening housing wealth inequalities as a prime example (Shelter, 2005). At the time of the status report's release, it was argued that, rather than focusing on changing the 'health choices' of millions of individuals, the government should perhaps think more about a healthier way to govern – making the long overdue, but still salient, choices at its disposal to use the tax and benefit systems to kerb growing social inequalities and redistribute income and – *most importantly* – wealth (Shaw et al, 2005a, authors' italics). By 2005, of 26 countries in Europe only four had a higher rate of child poverty than the United Kingdom and only one recorded a higher rate before state transfers of benefits: the Slovak Republic (Hirsch, 2006). Under the first 10 years of the New Labour government, inequalities in mortality rates rose relentlessly. They did not do so under previous Old Labour administrations (Shaw et al, 1999).

## Conclusion

During his 'new thinking' lecture tour of 2006, the Prime Minister announced that public health problems were no longer public health problems (see also Chapters Four, Five, Eight, Nine and Eleven for further discussion of New Labour's shift to choice and individual responsibility in relation to health). This was an attempt to achieve for social medicine what Margaret Thatcher so famously tried for sociology when she said that there was no such thing as society. Tony Blair's exact words were: 'Our public health problems are not, strictly speaking, public health questions at all. They are questions of individual lifestyle – obesity, smoking, alcohol abuse, diabetes, sexually transmitted disease' (Blair, 2006). Within six weeks of making that claim, the Prime Minister was forced to announce that he would resign within the year, although his pillorying of public health may not have been at the forefront of any list of reasons suggested by those who forced his hand. He, and by implication much New Labour thinking, had clearly become part of the problem rather than part of the solution to reducing inequalities in health in Britain.

## References

Acheson, D. (1998) *Independent inquiry into inequalities in health*, London: The Stationery Office.

Berridge, V. (ed) (2002) 'The Black Report and the health divide', *Cont Br Hist*, vol 16, pp 131-71.

Black, D., Morris, N.J., Smith, C. and Townsend, P. (1999) 'Better benefits for health: plan to implement the central recommendation of the Acheson report', *BMJ*, vol 318, pp 724-7.

Blair, T. (2001) Interview with Jeremy Paxman on Newsnight (available at http://news.bbc.co.uk/hi/english/events/newsnight/newsid_1372000/1372220.stm).

Blair, T. (2006) 'Blair backs healthy living', 26 July (available at http://news.bbc.co.uk/1/hi/uk_politics/5215548.stm).

Davey Smith, G., Morris J, and Shaw, M. (1998) 'The independent inquiry into inequalities in health: a worthy successor to the Black Report?' *BMJ*, vol 317, pp 1465-6.

Davey Smith, G., Dorling, D., Gordon, D. and Shaw, M. (1999) 'The widening health gap: what are the solutions?', *Critical Public Health*, vol 9, no 2, pp 151-70.

Davey Smith, G., Dorling, D., Mitchell, R. and Shaw, M. (2002) 'Health inequalities in Britain: continuing increases up to the end of the 20th century', *Journal of Epidemiology and Community Health*, vol 56, pp 434-5.

DH (Department of Health) (1997) 'Public health strategy launched to tackle the root causes of ill health', Press release, 7 July.

DH (1998) *On the state of the public health 1997: The annual report of the Chief Medical Officer of the Department of Health for the year 1997,* London: The Stationery Office.

DH (2001) *Health inequalities: National targets on infant mortality and life expectancy – technical briefing* (revised 2002) (www.dh.gov.uk/assetRoot/04/07/78/96/04077896.pdf).

DH (2004) *Choosing health: Making healthy choices easier,* Cm 6374, London: Department of Health.

DH (2005a) *Tackling health inequalities: Status report on the Programme for Action,* London: Department of Health.

DH (2005b) *Health trainers for disadvantaged areas,* Press release, 11 August (www.dh.gov.uk/en/Publicationsandstatistics/Pressrelease/DH_4117720).

DHSS (Department of Health and Social Security) (1980) *Inequalities in health: Report of a research working group* (Black Report), London: DHSS.

DSS (Department of Social Security) (1998) *Households below average income 1979-1996,* London: The Stationery Office.

Dorling, D. (2005) *Human geography of the UK,* London: Sage Publications.

Dorling, D. (2006) 'Class alignment renewal', *The Journal of Labour Politics,* vol 14, no 1, pp 8-19.

Dorling, D., Eyre, H., Johnston, R. and Pattie, C. (2002) 'A good place to bury bad news? Hiding the detail in the geography on the Labour Party's website, reports and surveys', *The Political Quarterly,* vol 73, no 4, pp 476-92.

Dorling, D., Ford, J., Holmans, A., Sharp, C., Thomas, B. and Wilcox, S. (2005) *The great divide: An analysis of housing inequality,* London: Shelter.

Grice, A. (2001) 'Blair awards himself 41% pay increase', *The Independent,* 12 June.

*Hansard* (1997) House of Lords, 12 February, cols 248-9.

Hillyard, P., Pantazis, C., Tombs, S., Gordon, D. and Dorling, D. (2005) *Criminal obsessions: Why harm matters more than crime,* London: Pluto Press.

Hirsh, D. (2006) 'Why we are failing our children', *New Statesman,* 10 July, pp 10-17.

Howarth, C., Kenway, P., Palmer, G. and Street, C. (1998) *Key indicators of poverty and social exclusion,* York: Joseph Rowntree Foundation.

Lynch, J.W. and Kaplan, G.A. (1997) 'Understanding how inequality in the distribution of income affects health', *Journal of Health Psychology,* vol 2, pp 297-314.

Marmot, M. (2004) *Review 2004: Promoting medical science and its rapid translation into healthcare benefits for patients*, London: The Academy of Medical Sciences.

Marmot, M. (2005) Interview on the Today programme, BBC Radio 4, 12 August.

ONS (Office of National Statistics) (2005) 'Births, perinatal and infant mortality statistics, 2002' (www.statistics.gov.uk/STATBASE/Expodata/Spreadsheets/D6951.xls).

Shaw, M., Dorling, D., Gordon, D. and Davey Smith, G. (1999) *The widening gap: Health inequalities and policy in Britain*, Bristol: The Policy Press.

Shaw, M., Dorling, D., Mitchell, R. and Davey Smith, G. (2005a) 'Labour's "Black Report" moment', *BMJ*, vol 331, p 575.

Shaw, M., Davey Smith, G. and Dorling, D. (2005b) 'Health inequalities and New Labour: how the promises compare with real progress', *BMJ*, vol 330, pp 1016-21.

Shelter (2005) *The great divide: An analysis of housing inequality*, London: Shelter.

Townsend, P. and Davidson, N. (1982) *Inequalities in health: The Black Report*, Harmondsworth: Penguin.

Waugh, P. (1999) 'Pledge by PM to end child poverty', *The Independent*, 18 March.

Wintour, P. (2004) 'Inequality up under Labour', *The Guardian*, 3 August.

# FOUR

# Explaining inequalities in health: theoretical, conceptual and methodological agendas

*Simon J. Williams, Michael Calnan and Alan Dolan*

## Introduction

How are we to explain inequalities in health? Are some pathways more important than others? Are there limits to current epidemiological research? What light does lay knowledge shed on inequalities in health, both past and present? Do we need to dig deeper into the causes of inequalities? How do these issues translate into future policies and practices designed to tackle inequalities in health and 'narrow the gap'? These are some of the questions confronting health inequalities researchers today. The importance of these questions, moreover, seems to have grown rather than diminished in the light of the UK government White Paper for England (DH, 2004), tellingly entitled *Choosing health: Making healthier choices easier*: a side-stepping, effectively, of anything but behavioural/ lifestyle explanations, couched in the rhetoric of consumer choice.

Recent years have witnessed what might be termed a 'reinvigorated' debate around potential pathways and explanations for health inequalities, including the limits of epidemiological approaches and a reassessment of the role of different types of knowledge and expertise. Richard Wilkinson's work on income distribution and social relativities, in particular, has been an important influence here, both before and since the Acheson Inquiry (Acheson, 1998), generating much discussion and debate. It is with a detailed exposition of this discussion and debate, therefore, together with other new lines of thinking and research on inequalities in health, that this chapter is concerned. Following a brief account of Wilkinson's so-called 'psychosocial' perspective on income distribution, social relativities and health, we then proceed to discuss recent research on lay knowledge and life-course approaches respectively. We also return, towards the end of the chapter, to some further thoughts and reflections on *Choosing health* in the light of these debates, paying particular attention to future research and policy agendas for tackling health inequalities and reducing 'the gap'. While *Choosing health* is very much an English public health White Paper, analysis of Scottish and Welsh health documents (Raphael and Bryant, 2006) highlights a similar emphasis on a behavioural/lifestyle approach to improving inequalities in health (see Scottish Executive, 2004; Welsh Assembly, 2004).

## The psychosocial perspective

Since the Black Report (DHSS, 1980) presented its findings, scepticism has grown as to the explanatory power of its materialist explanations for inequalities in health. What might be termed the 'direct' effects of material living standards, such as poor housing conditions, environmental pollution and employment in the heaviest and most hazardous industries, are well-established causes of health inequalities. However, whereas 'traditional' material explanations contribute to our understanding of health inequalities between rich and poor, they are less able to account for the observed gradients in health and mortality that exist right across society (Bartley et al, 1998). Evidence shows that those at the top of the social hierarchy have better health than those close to the top, yet neither of these groups could be said to be disadvantaged in terms of standards of living. Moreover, evidence also shows that in Western societies, once a certain level of material wealth has been attained and the 'epidemiological transition' from infectious to chronic degenerative diseases completed, health is related less to overall wealth and more to how equally or unequally this wealth is distributed (Graham, 2001).

In recent years, a relative outpouring of research has sought to extend, refine and develop materialist explanations to account for contemporary links between social structure and health. Much of this attention has focused on the health-damaging effects of relative rather than absolute deprivation. Central to these developments has been a growing interest in psychosocial explanations, stimulated in the main by the research of Richard Wilkinson (1986, 1990, 1992, 1994a, 1994b, 1996, 2005), which has concentrated on the links between income inequality and life expectancy. As one of the leading proponents of psychosocial approaches to health inequalities, Wilkinson suggests that the main effects of living standards and social circumstances may not be directly due to material deprivation itself, but are mediated by psychological responses to relative deprivation and low social status, whatever the actual material conditions of life. This is not to suggest that psychosocial pathways are independent from material ones, but they are differentiated as being located in the social and economic problems that affect health 'indirectly' through various forms of worry, stress, insecurity and vulnerability. Wilkinson argues that these and other negative emotions are translated inside the body into poorer health, via the body's internal stress systems. In addition, increased levels of stress and other negative emotions may carry a further health penalty in terms of increasing the likelihood of risk-taking forms of behaviour. To substantiate his argument, Wilkinson provides impressive evidence of health-related physiological consequences of low social status from studies of non-human primates. While both the direct and indirect pathways are in operation as absolute deprivation is reduced, the psychosocial effects of relative deprivation become pre-eminent in the aetiology of ill health:

> When looking at the nature of the pathways which are most likely to link physical disease to inequality, there is good reason for thinking that psychosocial pathways are more important. Simply the fact that we are dealing with the effect of relative differences, rather than absolute material standards points strongly in that direction (Wilkinson, 1996, p 175).

Findings from the Whitehall II study of British civil servants shed further light on these 'biologically plausible ways' in which social experience – such as low control/high demands at work – 'translates' into disease (Marmot, 2004). Metabolic syndrome,[1] for example, was found to increase in frequency as hierarchy was descended: the lower the employment grade, the lower the HDL cholesterol, the higher the plasma triglycerides and the higher the fasting levels of glucose and insulin (Marmot, 2004, p 121).

Wilkinson's hypothesis not only accounts for the negative effects of the subjective experience of relative deprivation on individual health, but also addresses the impact of relative deprivation on more broadly based social processes significant for population health and life expectancy. As he clearly demonstrates, it is not the richest but the most egalitarian societies that have the best health, which he believes to be due to more equitable forms of income distribution that engender trust and result in more socially cohesive societies. They have larger amounts of what has been termed social capital: defined as 'networks, norms, and trust ... that enable participants to act together more effectively to pursue shared objectives' (Wilkinson, 1996, p 221, quoting

Putnam, 1995, pp 664-5). In contrast, countries such as Britain have experienced the damaging effects of an increasingly 'individualised' and unequal society, in terms of increasing numbers experiencing relative deprivation, which has exacerbated existing social divisions and made it more difficult to maintain communal bonds conducive to good health.

Wilkinson's work suggests that it is not so much the direct effects of absolute material living standards as the indirect effects of 'social relativities' that have most impact on health in modern Western societies. In his view, a sense of 'distributive justice' is the most important determinant of the psychosocial well-being of a society. Reducing the numbers in society experiencing relative deprivation, through a more equal distribution of income, therefore provides policy makers with a way of improving the health of the whole population, independent of an individual's relative position. In making the links between personal problems and the broader social structure, Wilkinson believes that the psychosocial perspective on health inequalities provides a more realistic assessment of the integration of the individual/biological and society and links population health more closely to wider social problems.

We are, according to Wilkinson, entering a new phase of 'integrative' thinking regarding inequalities in health, thanks to the promise and potential of the psychosocial perspective or approach. Psychosocial pathways, to repeat, are not independent of material ones. The psychosocial perspective, furthermore, provides the opportunity to integrate biological and social factors, to explore more fully the relationship between the individual and society and to link health inequalities to other social problems such as crime. Issues of gender, 'race' and inequality have also been more directly and explicitly addressed in Wilkinson's (2005) most recent work. Although more unequal societies are more male-dominated and the position of women deteriorates relative to men, men's death rates are nonetheless, Wilkinson notes, 'more adversely affected by inequality than women's' (p 215). Similarly, it is 'almost certainly true that social relations among men are more damaged by inequality than social relations among women' (2005, p 215). Men, in other words, appear to be 'harmed even more by male domination than women' (p 215). Why? Because inequality, in keeping with Wilkinson's general line of reasoning, 'increases status competition amongst men' (2005, p 215). There may, moreover, be important gender differences in psychosocial pathways to social inequality and disease. Recent findings from the Whitehall II study, for instance, show that low social control at home predicted heart disease in women, but not in men (Chandola et al, 2004).[2] The health of ethnic minorities also, of course, shows the 'heavy burden of their social and economic disadvantage' (p 216). Ethnicity, Wilkinson contends, 'becomes a mark of collective social status, and its inescapability increases its health impact. Most of the processes of racism and stigmatisation are likely to increase with increasing inequality' (2005, p 216).[3] A particularly interesting concept in this respect, borrowed from Adorno's *The authoritarian personality* (Adorno et al, 1950), is the 'bicycling reaction' in which 'increased inequality and dominance relations lead to more discrimination against any vulnerable group, including ethnic minorities' (Wilkinson, 2005, p 224). These types of 'bicycling reaction', indeed, are most frequent in times of high unemployment and economic hardship 'when people feel their dignity and status is threatened by relative poverty' (Wilkinson, 2005, p 225).

Wilkinson's work then, as this suggests, provides an important new approach and perspective on inequalities with the self-professed promise and potential for new forms of 'integrative' thinking. But what, we might still legitimately ask, about lay knowledge/expertise? For all its promise and potential, the psychosocial perspective, as currently constituted, accords little room to lay perspectives and experience in helping us unravel the complexities of health inequalities, both past and present. It is to these very matters, therefore, that we now turn.

## Lay knowledge/expertise

The category of lay knowledge (Calnan, 1987) appears to have emerged when sociologists and anthropologists attempted to shift accounts of illness and health-related behaviour away from positivistic and individualistic explanations to those that have put an emphasis on the pluralistic and interpretative nature of the social world. Lay knowledge became embedded in the health inequalities debate when attempts were made to explain the possible link between social structure, beliefs and practices (Blaxter, 2004). These approaches attempted to give meaning to the adoption of 'risk-related' behaviours by people living in adverse social circumstances. For example, one type of approach focused on the way women bringing up children were constrained by adverse social and material circumstances in adopting their preferred health-related practices, for example patterns of food consumption or giving up smoking (Graham, 2001).

There was, however, as Prior points out (2003), an apparent shift over this period in the way the category of lay knowledge was conceptualised or formulated. Peoples' beliefs about cause shifted or evolved into the sturdier notion of lay knowledge, and lay concepts of aetiology and disease causation turned into a focus on lay epidemiology and the emergence of the notion of the 'lay' expert. 'A concern with belief had been transposed into a concern with knowledge and that lay people had metamorphosed into multi-skilled and knowledgeable individuals' (Prior, 2003, p 45). This apparent transition in the conceptualisation of lay knowledge is important as it can be used to make sense of more recent formulations and uses of 'lay knowledge'. For example, Williams and Popay (1994) draw attention to a local community's response to the effects on the local water supply of a mercury spillage as illustrative of how lay people, drawing on their own sources of epidemiological knowledge, contest official reports.

The significance of 'lay knowledge' in the context of the recent sociological analysis of health inequalities reflects dissatisfaction with the explanatory power of the social epidemiological or social model. Emphasis has been placed on the need to open up the 'black box' (Wainwright and Calnan, 2002; Williams, 2003) and particularly the need to understand the contextual processes whereby class and other elements of social structure unfold in human relations, affecting a range of 'outcomes', including health. Thus, there is a need to theorise the bridge between structure and agency. For Williams (2003), this analysis needs to include the notion of 'place'. The study of the places people inhabit may be a way of exploring the way in which structures work themselves through into the dynamics of everyday life. 'Places can be conceptualised as the locations for structuration – the interrelationship of the conscious intentions and actions of individuals and groups and the "environment" of cultural, social and economic forces in which people exist' (Popay et al, 1998, p 74). This analysis of place and more generally the analysis of agency and structure also, according to Williams (2003), needs to be informed by a robust, historical perspective that also takes biography into account. 'Places have different histories, and the history of a neighbourhood or locality will mean different things to individual people who have their own temporal and historical associations with the area' (Popay et al, 1998, p 75). This in turn brings into play the importance of 'causal' or 'knowledgeable' narratives that contextualise explanations and connect context to composition, places to people. These lay causal narratives help people construct a sense of identity and purpose when they are trying to manage life under difficult social and economic condition (Williams, 2003). Narrative identity and relational settings are believed to be the two essential components for the conceptual bridge between structure and agency (Popay et al, 1998), with relational settings being characterised as the relationship between people, narrative and institutions.

This theoretical bridge is illustrated through empirical research (Popay et al, 2003) that identifies an apparent contradiction in informants' accounts of inequalities in health. On the one hand, informants gave vivid accounts of how living in difficult places had negative effects on their health and the role of others. On the other hand, informants were reluctant to accept the notion of inequalities in health and between areas and social groups. This apparent contradiction is resolved through the informants' use of narrative constructions of moral and social identity in which strength of character and personal control are emphasised (Popay et al, 2003). This parallels the evidence from Cornwell's (1984) ethnography in East London, which showed that, while informants accepted that work and life opportunities were limited, they also asserted that it was necessary to do 'one's best' and not give up or be 'fatalistic'.

Informants in Popay and colleagues' (2003) study also showed that their causal narratives invoked psychosocial pathways to link material and health disadvantage. This mirrors the sociological discourse on inequalities. However, the 'lay discourse' from 20 years earlier (Calnan, 1987) emphasised the role of health services and the lack of access to private healthcare as the major reason for inequalities in health. The role of health services was prevalent in the sociological debate about inequalities in health in the 1980s but it is now absent and also appears to be absent from informants' accounts. Lay knowledge, in this respect, was portrayed as a source for constructing identity rather than as an expert source of knowledge that paralleled professional opinion.

Lay knowledge then, from this perspective, is central to understanding and explaining inequalities in health: a lived as well as a theoretical bridge between structure and agency, people and places, composition and context. A sociological approach to health inequalities, linking personal troubles to public issues of social structure (cf Mills, 1959) demands no less.

## Health across the life course: class, time and biography

Although not directly linked or related, this discussion of people and places raises further important questions about health, not simply at one point in time but across the life course. We can date the emergence of life-course perspectives and approaches to health inequalities from the early 1980s, as new data from longitudinal studies began to emerge and the limits of some of the older perspectives on health inequalities became increasingly apparent (see, for example, Power et al, 1991; Wadsworth, 1991). The general thrust of the life-course approaches and explanations, as the term suggests, is to introduce a temporal dimension into the analysis in terms of the accumulation of (dis)advantage throughout our lives, thereby helping bring past and present together, so to speak, in explaining health inequalities. The way is cleared, moreover, for tracing the role of different factors and processes in different diseases over time. There are, nonetheless, as Bartley (2004) notes, different strands of thinking within this so-called life-course approach. Thus, while some (early) approaches appear in large part to extend former indirect selection explanations by looking at past factors, such as educational attainment, that might help explain present health inequalities, other approaches, indebted to more biological explanations, have looked for certain 'critical periods' in time, even in utero, that place individuals at particular risk of health problems in later life. Other approaches, in contrast, have focused on the 'accumulation' of hazards and adverse events over time in a largely additive fashion. A further strand of thinking here focuses on 'interactions' between experiences, whereby certain adverse events only seem to affect health to the extent that they interact with previous exposures and experiences, thereby rendering individuals or particular groups of people vulnerable or susceptible to disease. Finally, we may mention approaches that look at 'pathways', whereby certain hazards are seen to increase the risk of disease due to their role in increasing the possibility of some other aetiological factor(s) (Bartley, 2004, p 104).

While these various strands of thinking are subject to ongoing debate, it is not, of course, necessary to choose between them. We may, instead, prefer to think in terms of various mixtures of these different processes over time. Bartley's own favoured resolution, indeed, is for something akin to a 'life course political economy' of health, which examines the 'ways in which economic and social policies influence the accumulation of material and psycho-social risk' (2004, p 115). The ways in which advantage and disadvantage combine over the life course, from this perspective, influence 'how long each individual may spend in good health, and also what form of illness they may acquire' (2004, p 115).

Blaxter (2000), too, in her own recent musings on class, time and health, provides some further promising leads here. A distinction is drawn in this respect between social time, calendar time, and personal or biographical time. Individuals, Blaxter notes, have their own definitions of biotemporal orderliness that provide structure to their life and death. One of the factors for those living in deprivation, for example, is that time accelerates the perceived ageing process and makes those in such circumstances feel deprived of time. More importantly, Blaxter (2003) suggests that thinking in terms of a 'health capital' model is a profitable way forward here. As a heuristic, it may serve to direct research towards dealing with the complexity of class-related patterns of health, anchoring explanations, at one and the same time, firmly in the body. As a model, it accommodates processes of time, both individual and societal, and both 'real' or biological, or as constructed by the individual. Its gain or loss is 'intimately connected with the mutual interplay of agency and structure across time. Health capital connects the different stages of life together, and the varying influences that bear upon health status at any point in time' (2003, pp 81-2). Seen in these terms, indeed, any debate about whether social status is 'psychologically referenced through stress, self-esteem, social dysfunction or distress, or socially referenced through income, occupation, housing, the physical environment, or work dangers, is unprofitable. Of course, the answer is both, and the body is the link and the boundary between them' (2003, p 82).

Life-course approaches and explanations, then, as this brief discussion attests, help overcome some of the limits of older perspectives on health inequalities, introducing an important temporal dimension or dynamic into the analysis, thereby bringing the past to bear on the present throughout the individual's lifetime. The tracing or tracking of different causal factors and processes for different diseases over time, moreover, adds a new layer of complexity and sophistication into the analysis. At one and the same time, it should be noted, work of this kind involves large-scale longitudinal data sets, underpinned by a positivist methodology, which again leaves little room for more nuanced qualitative data of the kind identified in the previous section of this chapter on lay knowledge/lay expertise. There is no easy or obvious way, moreover, as Bartley (2004, p 131) comments, of reconciling strict psychosocial and life-course approaches, given that the former tend to be primarily based on 'period effects' (that is, income inequality at a given point in time) and the latter on 'cohort' effects (that is, things that happen to groups of people born at a given point in time). Bartley's own 'life-course political economy' approach and Blaxter's 'health capital' model, to be sure, go some way towards addressing these problems, but we may also need to dig much 'deeper', so to speak, if we are to truly understand and explain the nature and dynamics of health inequalities, both past and present.

## 'Digging deeper': neo-liberalism, class relations and capital flows

It is at this point that a further set of pertinent questions arises, namely, whether or not we need to 'dig deeper' into the causes of inequalities, and if so, where exactly we should be looking or digging. In part, of course, this returns us to the limits of neo-positivist, epidemiological, 'black box' research – where social processes are reduced to quantifiable variables – and to recent neo-materialist critiques of psychosocial explanations based on income inequalities (cf Muntaner and Lynch, 1999; Lynch et al, 2000). It also, however, adds important new dimensions to these debates that take us far beyond these earlier approaches and perspectives.

Coburn (2000a, 2000b, 2004), for example, in a series of papers, has highlighted the important role that neo-liberalism plays as the explanatory factor behind income inequality, social cohesion and the health status of populations. Wilkinson's work in particular, and the neo-positivist research on health inequalities in general, is again taken to task here for abandoning the search for causes and underlying generative mechanisms too soon. Not enough attention, that is to say, has been paid to the social context of factors such as income inequality. It is not so much a question, from this perspective, of income inequality leading to low social cohesion and poor health status, but of neo-liberalism – defined, broadly speaking, as a more or less thorough adherence to a market-oriented society – producing 'both higher income inequality and lower social cohesion and, presumably, either lowered health status or a health status which is not as high as it might otherwise have been' (Coburn, 2000a, p 137). The rise of neo-liberalism and the decline of the welfare state, in turn, are tied to processes of globalisation (that is, global competition and the mobility of capital) and the changing class structure of advanced capitalist societies. More attention, therefore, in Coburn's view, needs to be paid to understanding the 'causes of income inequalities' rather than just their 'effects' (2000a, p 135). The 'rise' and 'fall' of the welfare state, not least the 'privatisation' of the NHS by stealth (cf Pollock, 2004), together with the presumed class causes and consequences of these relations, are thereby drawn 'back in' to the analysis, with important implications for the causal pathways involved in income inequality–health status relationships and vice versa (Coburn, 2000a, p 137). The benefits of public systems of health and welfare for creating social cohesion and including all income groups are also thrown into critical relief.

The argument here is broadly realist in tone and content, critical realist in fact: a distinctly post-positivist position within the inequalities in health debate, centred on a reinvigorated class agenda. A realist approach to explaining inequalities, Scambler (2002, 2005) argues, deals with the deeper relations and generative mechanisms of class that are 'real', even if they are not directly observable, empirically speaking. We need, that is to say, to go beyond the surface and to take class, as well as gender and ethnicity, seriously rather than treating them as mere variables. Once this is done, it brings into play related sociological questions about where wealth and power go. Significant social change, from this perspective, has indeed occurred, yet class relations have remained: objectively they have become more salient while subjectively they play less of a role. We need to be alive, in other words, to continuities as well as discontinuities in the study of class relations over time.

Critical realism, in this respect, helps us to move 'back' or 'go beyond' income inequalities, and to reconceptualise class, as well as gender and ethnicity, in a more satisfactory sociological manner. Doing so, moreover, helps us reconceptualise former epidemiological variables in terms of capital, or flows of capital, over the life course, including not only material capital, but also biological capital, psychological capital, cultural capital, spatial capital, and perhaps even emotional capital. Relations of class, for example, greatly affect flows to individuals of these different types of capital over the life course, with the potential to have an impact on health and longevity.

As for sociology's own role within all this, it may very well be the case, as Scambler (2005) argues, not simply of a 'useful' (that is, applied policy-relevant) sociology of health inequalities, but also of something akin to a 'useless' sociology (in current policy terms at least) that maintains an 'outsider' stance and continues to focus on awkward or uncomfortable questions of wealth and power, thereby helping us to fully appreciate the generative mechanisms underpinning continuing inequalities in health that government and policy makers find difficult to address. There are, as this suggests, more theoretically justifiable ways of doing sociological research on health inequalities, in which questions of who owns what, and who has the power to do what, loom large.

There are echoes here, to be sure, with what Burawoy (2005) has usefully termed 'critical' sociology and 'public' sociology (as opposed to 'professional' sociology and 'policy' sociology). While a critical sociology, in this respect, draws attention to the limits and problems of existing research and policy on inequalities in health to date – including the norms, values and assumptions underpinning it and the power relations within which it is embedded – a public sociology seeks to reinvigorate the public sphere through renewed dialogue and democratic debate, thereby providing an important and powerful means through which governments may be held to account (see Chapter Three of this volume). A critical sociology, in short, is the 'conscience' of professional sociology, just as a public sociology is the conscience of policy sociology.[4]

## Health as choice or health as right: the slide into consumerism

What light, then, does the foregoing discussion of various perspectives and positions in the inequalities in health debate cast on the government White Paper *Choosing health: Making healthier choices easier* (DH, 2004)?

In contrast to the preceding governments of the 1980s and 1990s, New Labour came to power in 1997 seemingly impatient to translate the evidence on health inequalities accumulated since the publication of the Black Report into policy action. Among the aims set out in its first White Paper on public health, *Saving lives: Our healthier nation*, published in July 1999, were improvements in the health of the population generally, particularly those worst off, and the narrowing of the health gap between rich and poor (DH, 1999). In setting out its blueprint for tackling health inequalities, the White Paper made explicit reference to the role of material circumstances in the aetiology of ill health – 'widespread' inequalities resulted in the disadvantaged having 'suffered the most from poor health' – while noting that people could 'make individual decisions about their own and their families' health which can make a difference' (1999, p 3). The White Paper, as such, was acknowledged as evidence of the government's attention to the wider social and structural determinants of health. Concerns were raised, nonetheless, about the lack of targets for reducing health inequalities and whether or not government policies would be effective in achieving their goal of reducing inequalities in health (Shaw et al, 1998). Calls for the government to adopt policies that reduce poverty and income inequality as the most effective means of tackling health inequalities have also been largely ignored.

As for New Labour's latest White Paper on public health, *Choosing health: Making healthier choices easier*, this certainly represents a shift, albeit a regressive one, in the government's approach to tackling health inequalities, enshrining a renewed emphasis on the importance of health promotion strategies to inform individuals about lifestyle choices associated with good health. Exploring the precedents underlying this reversal in policy, Hunter (2005) draws attention to two earlier health reports produced by Derek Wanless, a former banker and special adviser to the Treasury. The first report (Wanless, 2002) presented his assessment of the resources necessary to provide high-quality health services in the future. Significantly, it concluded that the extent to which substantially increased investment in healthcare would lead to large health gains was dependent on how well people became 'fully engaged' with their own health, that is, the ability of individuals to take greater responsibility for their health. With this in mind, the report recommended investment in reducing demand by enhancing the promotion of good health and disease prevention.

Wanless developed these views in his second report, *Securing good health for the whole population*, published in 2004, which set out to review public health policy and assess progress in implementing the fully engaged scenario for health. The report was critical of the long-term failure of policy to shift the NHS from an acute service to one that promoted the maintenance of good health. Allied to this, it pointed to a disjointed and thinly spread public health workforce that lacked capacity to pursue an effective fully engaged health agenda. There was no single, easily accessible source of health advice for concerned individuals, for example. To assist the full engagement of the population, Wanless articulated the need for interventions to raise levels of health literacy among the public:

> Individuals are ultimately responsible for their own and their children's health and it is the aggregate actions of individuals which will ultimately be responsible for whether or not such an optimistic scenario as 'fully engaged' unfolds. People need to be supported more actively to make better decisions about their own health and welfare because there are widespread, systematic failures that influence the decisions individuals currently make. (Wanless, 2004, p 4).

This approach is entirely consistent with the philosophy underlying the new White Paper, *Choosing health*, which aims to support individuals to make informed choices about their health. Although the White Paper continues to acknowledge the 'need to focus specifically on tackling inequalities in health' (DH, 2004, p 10), this is not one of the three core principles – 'informed choice', 'personalisation' and 'working together' – that will underpin future attempts to narrow the widening health gap. In other words, the government now aims to reduce health inequalities not by tackling the wider determinants of health, but by promoting choice: 'Our fundamental aim must be to create a society where more people, particularly those in disadvantaged groups and poor areas, are encouraged and enabled to make healthier choices' (DH, 2004, p 11). To the extent that the core principles of the White Paper centre on 'informed choice', 'personalisation' and 'working together', it is clearly heavily indebted to the behavioural/lifestyle school of thought – including the advent of NHS health trainers and personal health kits – that both Acheson and Black before it largely rejected. The government's fear or even phobia of turning Britain into a nanny state, in this respect, and its commitment to health in consumer society, seems to have resulted in a confused or confusing and incomplete picture: one circumscribed by consumerism and individualism and limited, mainly, to avoidable chronic diseases (Rayner, 2004).

The White Paper, moreover, is replete with references to 'public consultation', 'reconnecting with people's lives', 'working together', 'effective partnerships' , 'community-based models for improving local health', and the provision of 'collective support' to help create an environment that 'promotes healthy choices'. The fact remains, nonetheless, that people are not competing on a level playing field when it comes the drivers or social determinants of health, let alone consumerism (Rayner, 2004). Informed choice, to be sure, is important. However, for many people, particularly those in disadvantaged circumstances, health is 'no more a matter of individual choice than the weather' (UKPHA, 2005, p 6). If 'choice' is the order of the day, in other words, deprived groups are doubly disadvantaged, given that they lack the resources necessary to exercise it.

Taken together, the explanations for inequalities in health considered in this chapter provide a powerful reminder of the limits of any such government public health programme. At most, the White Paper represents a retreat or slipping back into a behavioural/lifestyle diagnosis or explanation of the problem, and a nod in the direction of listening to local voices and working with local communities in order to make healthier choices, emphasis on choices, easier. The importance of tackling income inequalities, in this respect, drops out of the picture altogether, as do the deeper social drivers of inequality. Instead of opposing anti-health forces, or the manufacturers of ill health, through legislative action and the like, the new public health strategy aims to work with them (in the main) through voluntary agreements with the threat of legislation later. Why wait? Whatever happened, moreover, to health as a citizenship right rather than a consumer choice? Viewed in this light, then, the White Paper is not simply a betrayal of the Acheson

Inquiry, but also of the Black Report before it; a shift, in effect, from a public to a private conception of public health (cf Hunter, 2005).

So why this change of heart or direction on the part of New Labour? Why has New Labour dropped its stance on social capital and communitarian values, and shifted towards choice and the marketisation of healthcare? Has there been a shift in values or is it just a pragmatic policy in which nothing much has changed? One may very well point, as Hunter (2005) rightly does, to Wanless's two seminal reports, and to New Labour's own 'quiet revolution' in the NHS – market-style incentives and competitive behaviours that trumped anything contemplated by the previous Conservatives' internal market reforms of the early 1990s – both of which required, if not necessitated, the 'updating' of the 1999 public health statement (*Saving lives: Our healthier nation*) in order to bring it into line with current government thinking on the importance of 'choice' and 'individualism', combined with market incentives to modify lifestyles (Hunter, 2005, p 1010). But here, once more, we need to dig deeper into the underlying drivers or mechanisms of the significant policy shifts themselves. And again, we venture, it is neo-liberalism and global capitalism that provide the answers, shifting and shaping not simply health inequalities themselves but the very policies (or perhaps, more correctly, the lack of effective policies) designed to tackle them. We are, in short, in the corporate global era of the 'captive state' (cf Monbiot, 2001).

## Conclusion: future research agendas

The main conclusions to be drawn from this chapter can be summarised as follows.

First, the need to focus on both macro and micro social relations in understanding and explaining health inequalities, and to move towards a more integrated phase of research, given the complex, multidimensional nature of health inequalities. Life-course perspectives and approaches, as we have seen, particularly a 'life-course political economy' of health (cf Bartley, 2004), have much to offer here, not least in adding an important temporal dimension into inequalities research and in tracing the role of different factors involved in different diseases. We should not, however, rest content here, or call the explanatory programme off too soon.

Second, following directly on from this first point, lay knowledge is a crucial part of this picture, helping us elucidate the historical relationship between people and places – what it is like to live here, for example, how things have changed over time, what has happened to these people over time (Williams, 2003).

Third, lay knowledge is also vital to the policy-making process. In particular, there is an urgent need to challenge or at least rethink the legitimacy of different types of 'evidence' (that is, what 'counts' in policy-making circles), given the dominance of so-called 'hard' quantitative research evidence, and to value experiential forms of knowledge/expertise, thereby giving people a voice in the policy-making process and helping forge 'bottom-up' rather than 'top-down' policies that do not simply problematise or blame individuals and communities.

Fourth, and perhaps most importantly, we should not lose sight of the 'bigger picture', including the need to go 'deeper' into the causes as well as the consequences of inequalities, including 'distal' links that individuals may or may not be aware of, and the need to explore more fully the role of factors such as neo-liberalism, global capitalism and so on. Thinking in terms of capital flows, moreover, is a useful way of conceptualising these issues across the life course.

As for sociology's role within all this, since this is the perspective from which we, the authors, write, a range of options or positions suggest themselves, from applied policy-focused research to broader, more critical work on issues of power, capital and the deeper drivers of inequalities in health; a 'reinvigorated' research agenda, in effect, that may or may not sit easily with current policy concerns and options. Both 'critical' and 'public' sociology, in this respect, have vital roles to play, not simply in facilitating and engendering democratic debate and reinvigorating the public sphere, but also, most importantly, in holding governments to account.

It is against this backdrop that the most recent government White Paper on public health must be evaluated, not least the readiness or willingness, let alone the ability in the global era, to take on entrenched powerful corporate interests whose prime concern is the making of healthy profits rather than healthy people. Here again we return to the role of neo-liberalism and the deeper drivers of inequalities in health, which extend far beyond any simple question or matter of individual qua consumer 'choice'. Public health, in short, cannot and should not become a 'private' matter.

## Notes

[1] Metabolic syndrome is characterised by central adiposity (that is, fat around the abdomen rather than the hips), lower levels of the 'good' HDL cholesterol, high levels of blood glucose and insulin in the fasting state, high levels of plasma triglycerides and high blood pressure (Marmot, 2004, p 118).

[2] For a fuller, more detailed account of the complexities of gender inequalities in health, and the conceptual, theoretical and methodological challenges of research in this area, see, for example, Annandale and Hunt (2000).

[3] For a more detailed account of the complexities of ethnic inequalities in health and the conceptual, theoretical and methodological challenges of research in this area, see Nazroo (2001), Karlsen and Nazroo (2001), and Chapter Six in this volume.

[4] The raison d'être of policy sociology, for Burawoy (2005), is to provide solutions to problems already defined and identified, or to legitimate solutions that have already been reached by client groups or policy makers. There can be neither policy nor public sociology, however, without a professional sociology that supplies tried and trusted methods, accumulated bodies of knowledge, orienting questions and conceptual frameworks. Professional sociology, indeed, is not the enemy of policy and public sociology but the '*sine qua non* of their existence', providing both legitimacy and expertise for policy and public sociology (2005, p 267). In practice, moreover, as Burawoy readily acknowledges, the boundaries between these ideal types of sociology are often blurred. Sociologists, for example, can and often do simultaneously serve a client (policy sociology) and generate debate (public sociology). For further lively debates on the role of sociology in relation to policy, see Johnson, 2004; Lauder et al, 2004; Wiles, 2004.

## References

Acheson, D. (1998) *Independent inquiry into inequalities in health*, London: The Stationery Office.

Adorno, T.W., Frenkel-Brunswik, E., Levinson, D.J. and Sanford, R.N. (1950) *The authoritarian personality*, New York: Harper.

Annandale, E. and Hunt, K. (eds) (2000) *Gender inequalities in health*, Buckingham: Open University Press.

Bartley, M. (2004) *Health inequalities: An introduction to theories, concepts and methods*, Cambridge: Polity Press.

Bartley, M., Blane, D. and Davey Smith, G. (1998) 'Introduction: beyond the Black Report', *Sociology of Health and Illness*, vol 20, no 5, pp 563-77.

Blaxter, M. (2000) 'Class, time and biography', in S.J. Williams, J. Gabe and M. Calnan (eds) *Health, medicine and society: Key theories, future agendas*, London: Routledge, pp 27-50.

Blaxter, M. (2003) 'Biology, social class and health inequalities: their synthesis in "health capital"', in S.J.Williams, L. Birke and G. Bendelow (eds) *Debating biology: Sociological reflections on health, medicine and society*, London: Routledge, pp 69-83.

Blaxter, M. (2004) *Health*, Cambridge: Polity Press.

Burawoy, M. (2005) 'American Sociological Association Presidential address: For Public Sociology', *British Journal of Sociology*, vol 56, no 2, pp 259-94.

Calnan, M. (1987) *Health and illness: The lay perspective*, London: Tavistock.

Chandola, T., Kuper, H., Singh-Manoux, M., Bartley, M. and Marmot, M. (2004) 'The effects of control at home on CHD events in the Whitehall II study: gender differences in psychosocial domestic pathways to social inequalities in CHD', *Social Science and Medicine*, vol 58, no 8, pp 1501-9.

Coburn, D. (2000a) 'Income inequality, social cohesion and the health status of populations: the role of neoliberalism', *Social Science and Medicine*, vol 51, no 1, pp 135-46.

Coburn, D. (2000b) 'A brief response', *Social Science and Medicine*, vol 51, no 7, pp 1009-10.

Coburn, D. (2004) 'Beyond the income inequality hypothesis: class, neo-liberalism and health inequalities', *Social Science and Medicine*, vol 58, no 1, pp 41-56.

Cornwell, J. (1984) *Hard-earned lives*, London: Tavistock.

DH (Department of Health) (1999) *Saving lives: Our healthier nation*, Cm 4386, London: The Stationery Office.

DH (2004) *Choosing health: Making healthier choices easier*, Cm 6374, London: The Stationery Office.

DHSS (Department of Health and Social Security) (1980) *Inequalities in health: Report of a research working group* (Black Report), London: DHSS.

Graham, H. (2001) 'The challenge of health inequalities', in H. Graham (ed) *Understanding health inequalities*. Buckingham: Open University Press, pp 1-24.

Hunter, D.J. (2005) 'Choosing or losing health?', *Journal of Epidemiology and Community Health*, vol 59, no 12, pp 1010-13.

Johnson, P (2004) 'Making social science useful', *British Journal of Sociology*, vol 55, no 1, pp 23-30.

Karlsen, S. and Nazroo, J. (2001) 'Identity and structure: rethinking ethnic inequalities in health', in H. Graham (ed) *Understanding health inequalities*, Buckingham: Open University Press, pp 38-57.

Lauder, H., Brown, P. and Halsey, A.H. (2004) 'Sociology and political arithmetic: some principles of a new policy science', *British Journal of Sociology*, vol 55, no 1, pp 3-22.

Lynch, J.W., Davey Smith, G., Kaplan, G.A. and House, J.S. (2000) 'Income inequality and mortality: importance to health of individual income, psychosocial environment, or material conditions', *BMJ*, vol 320, pp 1200-4.

Marmot, M. (2004) *Status syndrome*, London: Bloomsbury.

Mills, C.W. (1959) *The sociological imagination*, New York, NY: Oxford University Press.

Monbiot, G. (2001) *The captive state*, London: Pan.

Muntaner, C. and Lynch, J. (1999) 'Income inequality, social cohesion, and class relations: a critique of Wilkinson's neo-Durkheimian research programme', *International Journal of Health Services*, vol 29, no 1, pp 59-81.

Nazroo, J. (2001) *Ethnicity, class and health*, London: Policy Studies Institute.

Pollock, A.M. (2004) *NHS plc*, London: Verso.

Popay, J., Williams, G., Thomas, C. and Gatrell, A. (1998) 'Theorising inequalities in health: the place of lay knowledge', in M. Bartley, D. Blane and G. Davey Smith (eds) *Sociology of health inequalities*, Oxford: Blackwell Publishing, pp 59-84.

Popay, J., Bennett, S., Thomas, C., Williams, G., Gatrell, A. and Bostock, L. (2003) 'Beyond beer, fags, egg and chips? Exploring lay understanding of social inequalities in health', *Sociology of Health and Illness*, vol 25, no 1, pp 1-23.

Power, C., Manor, O. and Fox, J. (1991) *Health and class: The early years*, London: Chapman and Hall.

Prior, L. (2003) 'Belief, knowledge and expertise: the emergence of the lay expert in medical sociology', *Sociology of Health and Illness*, vol 25 (silver anniversary issue), pp 41-7.

Putnam, R.D. (1995) 'Tuning in, tuning out: the strange disappearance of social capital in America', *Political Science and Politics*, vol 28, no 4, pp 664-83.

Raphael, D. and Bryant, T. (2006) 'The state's role in promoting population health: Public health concerns in Canada, USA, UK, and Sweden', *Health Policy*, vol 78, no 1, pp 39-55.

Rayner, G. (2004) 'Choosing health: a policy fit for Bridget Jones?', *Public Health News*, 22 November, pp 10-11.

Scambler, G. (2002) *Health and social change: A critical theory*, Buckingham: Open University Press.

Scambler, G. (2005) 'Social structure and health: a narrative of neglect?' *Medical Sociology News*, vol 31, no 3, pp 53-69.

Scottish Executive (2004) *Improving health in Scotland*, Edinburgh: Scottish Executive.

Shaw, M., Dorling, D. and Davey Smith, G. (1999) *The widening gap: Inequalities in health in Britain*, Bristol: The Policy Press.

UKPHA (UK Public Health Association) (2005) *Choosing health or losing health? UK Public Health Association response to the White Paper 'Choosing health: Making healthier choices easier'*, London: UKPHA.

Wadsworth, M.E.J. (1991) *The imprint of time*, Oxford: Oxford University Press.

Wainwright, D. and Calnan, M. (2002) *Work stress: The making of an epidemic*, Basingstoke: Open University Press.

Wanless, D. (2002) *Securing our future health: Taking a long-term view. Final report*, London: HM Treasury (www.hm-treasury.gov.uk/consultations_and_legislation/wanless/consult_wanless_final.cfm).

Wanless, D. (2004) *Securing good health for the whole population. Final report*, London: HMSO (www.hm-treasury.gov.uk/consultations_and_legislation/wanless/consult_wanless04_final.cfm).

Welsh Assembly (2004) *Health challenge Wales*, Cardiff: Welsh Assembly.

Wiles, P. (2004) 'Policy and sociology', *British Journal of Sociology*, vol 55, no 1, pp 31-4.

Wilkinson, R.G. (1986) 'Income and mortality', in R.G. Wilkinson (ed) *Class and health: Research and longitudinal data*, London: Tavistock, pp 88-114.

Wilkinson, R.G. (1990) 'Income distribution and mortality: a "natural" experiment', *Sociology of Health and Illness*, vol 12, no 4, pp 391-411.

Wilkinson, R.G. (1992) 'Income distribution and life expectancy', *BMJ*, vol 304, pp 165-8.

Wilkinson, R.G. (1994a) 'Health, redistribution and growth', in A. Glyn and D. Miliband (eds) *Paying for inequality: The economic cost of social injustice*, London: Rivers Oram Press, pp 24-43.

Wilkinson, R.G. (1994b) *Unfair shares: The effects of widening income differentials on the welfare of the young*, Ilford: Barnardos.

Wilkinson, R.G. (1996) *Unhealthy societies: The afflictions of inequality*, London: Routledge.

Wilkinson, R.G. (2005) *The impact of inequality: How to make sick societies healthier*, London: Routledge.

Williams, G.H. (2003) 'The determinants of health: structure, context and agency', *Sociology of Health and Illness*, vol 25 (silver anniversary issue), pp 131-54.

Williams, G.H. and Popay, J. (1994) 'Researching the people's health: dilemmas and opportunities for social scientists', in Popay, J. and Williams, G.H. (eds) *Researching the people's health*, London: Routledge.

# FIVE

# Inequalities in pregnancy and early years and the impact across the life course: progress and future challenges

*Nick Spencer and Catherine Law*

## Introduction

Pregnancy and early childhood are particularly vulnerable stages in the life course at which adverse socioeconomic circumstances have lasting effects. Inequalities at this early stage of life have been shown to impact on adult health (Hertzman et al, 2001; Jefferis et al, 2002; Spencer, 2003) but they are also themselves the result of intergenerational inequalities (Spencer, 2004; Kahn et al, 2005). For infants surviving the first year of life, the effects of adverse pregnancy outcomes track into early childhood to contribute to inequalities in early childhood health (Pharoah et al, 1994; Jefferis et al, 2002) and form the early components of pathways that lead to health inequalities in adult life (Bartley et al, 1994; Power and Hertzman, 1999; Hertzman et al, 2001).

The Acheson Inquiry (Acheson, 1998) recognised the importance of health inequalities in pregnancy and early childhood both for infants and children themselves and for future adults, stating:

> We take the view that, while there are many potentially beneficial interventions to reduce inequalities in health in adults of working age and older people, many of those with the best chance of reducing future inequalities in mental and physical health relate to parents, particularly present and future mothers, and children. (p 9)

As the above quote suggests, reducing health inequalities at this critical point is vital to disrupting the intergenerational and individual life-course pathways that generate and sustain health inequalities across the life course. The New Labour government accepted the conclusions of the Acheson Inquiry and set in place policies to tackle inequalities (DH, 2003). For the first time, a UK government gave priority to reduction of health inequalities, instituting policies across government departments. The government also made improving the lives of children an explicit priority, exemplified by the Prime Minister's pledge to eliminate child poverty by 2020 (Blair, 1999).

This chapter aims to examine progress towards the goal of reducing pregnancy and early childhood inequalities since 1997 and outline future challenges. The chapter starts with a brief summary of inequalities in pregnancy and early childhood health, and inequalities in health determinants and their respective trends. We also consider the impact of the socioeconomic environment in childhood on health outcomes in later life. Policy initiatives since 1997 aimed at reducing these inequalities are outlined, along with an examination of the evidence for their effectiveness. Finally, future challenges and policy directions are discussed. The chapter is concerned primarily with UK children under five years of age, although comparative data from other countries are cited where appropriate. Policy differs in the four nations of the UK in some respects. Where relevant, the chapter will distinguish between policies as they apply to the four nations of the UK.

## Health inequalities in pregnancy and early childhood
### Inequalities in health outcomes

Inequalities in pregnancy complications and maternal mortality in developed countries have been less widely studied than inequalities in pregnancy outcomes. Maternal mortality is associated with social disadvantage and with being a lone parent, but there are now relatively small numbers of maternal deaths for analysis in many developed countries (CEMACH, 2004). A higher risk of maternal anaemia, infection, and premature rupture of membranes in low- compared with high-income mothers has been reported (Gudmundsson et al, 1997; Ferguson et al, 2002). Folate deficiency in pregnancy is socially patterned (James et al, 1997) and there is some evidence that its adverse effects on the growing fetus might be exacerbated by smoking (Relton et al, 2005).

Impaired fetal growth, in extreme form known as intrauterine growth retardation, is associated with adverse pregnancy outcomes (Pallotto and Kilbride, 2006) and with increased risk of some adverse adult health outcomes (Barker, 1998; Ben-Shlomo and Kuh, 2002). Impaired fetal growth is strongly socially patterned (Kramer et al, 2000).

Spontaneous abortion has been shown to be associated with lower occupation and social class among Finnish women (Hemminki et al, 1980). Stillbirth was 30% more likely in deprived compared with affluent areas of England and Wales (1986-92) although data from Cumbria covering a similar time period (1986-93) failed to show a significant difference in stillbirths by social group (Dummer et al, 2000). Perinatal mortality due to antenatal events had an 80% higher risk in the most - compared with the least – deprived quintile in the West Midlands region of the UK in 1991-93 (Bambang et al, 2000). The same study reported a twofold increase in perinatal deaths associated with congenital anomalies in the most – compared with the least – deprived quintile.

Socially disadvantaged infants are almost twice as likely to die in infancy compared with their more privileged peers (Drever and Whitehead, 1997). Social inequalities in deaths in the post-neonatal period (one to 12 months of age) are more marked than in the neonatal period (Maher and Macfarlane, 2004). Social inequalities in birth-weight have been extensively studied (see Spencer, 2003 for a detailed review of these studies) and these studies consistently show differences in mean birth-weight between the most privileged and the most disadvantaged of between 150 and 200g. Although the determinants vary over time and place (Fairley, 2005), higher social status appears to protect against low birth-weight. Preterm birth (<37 weeks' gestation) is associated with an increased risk of neonatal and early infancy morbidity and mortality and poorer mothers are more likely to give birth before term (Kramer et al, 2000; Ponce et al, 2005; Fairley and Leyland, 2006). A range of other adverse neonatal outcomes such as congenital anomalies and hypoglycaemia are also strongly socially patterned (Manning et al, 2005).

Cerebral palsy is the most common childhood physical disability. Inequalities in rates of cerebral palsy have been reported in studies from Ireland (Dowding and Barry, 1990) and the UK (Dolk et al, 2001; Sundrum et al, 2005). Inequalities in long-standing illness become established in early childhood (Spencer and Coe, 2003a). Non-accidental injury and child abuse are important causes of death and morbidity in early childhood (UNICEF, 2003). Studies based on child protection registration consistently show a social gradient in child maltreatment (Baldwin and Spencer, 1999; Sidebotham and Heron, 2006) but they may be subject to bias as child protection registration is itself socially patterned. However, in a study of young people aged

18-24 years in the UK, those from poorer homes were more likely to report experiencing non-accidental injury in their early childhood (Cawson et al, 2000). After the first year of life, unintentional injuries are the most important cause of mortality and morbidity in childhood and studies consistently show a marked social gradient (Laflamme and Diderichsen, 2000; Kendrick and Marsh, 2001).

Immunisation rates are also socially patterned, with lower rates of uptake in areas of high deprivation (Li and Taylor, 1993; Wright and Polack, 2006), although highly educated mothers are also less likely to have their babies immunised than those with lower educational attainment (Li and Taylor, 1993; Samad et al, 2006)

Mental health problems in childhood are recognised as a common cause of functional disability at all ages of childhood (Woodroffe et al, 1993). Poorer children are more likely to suffer behavioural and emotional problems throughout childhood (Meltzer et al, 2000) and inequalities in these conditions become established by the age of three years (Spencer and Coe, 2003b).

Thus, social inequalities in clinically important, common adverse pregnancy and early childhood health outcomes are well recognised in the UK and have a profound effect on population health.

## Inequalities in health determinants

Underpinning many of the inequalities in health outcomes outlined above are inequalities in those factors that determine health outcomes. Inequalities in some of the key determinants, such as smoking (see Chapter Nine of this volume), nutrition (Chapter Eight), housing (Chapter Seven) and ethnicity/racism (Chapter Six), are considered in detail in other chapters. These factors play an important role in relation to health inequalities in pregnancy and early childhood. For example, the marked social gradient in smoking in pregnancy is a major determinant of impaired fetal growth (Kramer et al, 2000) and the social gradient in breastfeeding contributes to higher rates of illness in early childhood among children in low-income families (Quigley et al, 2006).

Income operates as a background factor, exerting its influence through other determinants such as housing, nutrition and education. Low income appears to have a pervasive effect on health in pregnancy and early childhood that tracks into adulthood (see below). Families with young children in the UK are more likely to experience low income and this applies particularly to lone-parent families (DWP, 2005). Families with no working adult, families with a disabled adult or child, and those of Pakistani and Bangladeshi origin, are much more likely than other families to experience low income (DWP, 2005). Family income varies across time and children in families that are poor for longer periods are more likely to experience poor living conditions and have less access to a range of consumer goods than non-poor children and children who are only poor for short periods (Adelman et al, 2003).

Education, which is closely linked to income in many countries and particularly in the UK (Chevalier et al, 2005; Webber and Butler, 2006), impacts on health through other mediating variables. Maternal education, long recognised as a key variable in relation to child health (Caldwell, 1979), seems to protect children against poor health outcomes, but its impact may not be independent of income (Séguin et al, 2005). Higher levels of maternal education are associated with lower levels of household smoking and, hence, lower levels of infant exposure to tobacco smoke (Blackburn et al, 2003). Higher maternal education is also linked to breastfeeding in the UK (Papadimitriou et al, 2005).

Changing family structure, particularly the increase in lone-parent families, has been implicated in the increase in health inequalities as lone parents are both more likely to live in poor socioeconomic conditions and to have children with poorer health outcomes. In all rich nations, children of lone parents are more likely to live in poverty (UNICEF, 2001). Lone parenthood is associated with greater risk of poor pregnancy and early childhood outcomes but there is some evidence, at least from the UK, that this may be largely due to material disadvantage (Spencer, 2005).

In almost all societies, primary carers of infants and children are parents and, despite changes in family structure, most children in the UK are cared for by at least one of their biological parents. Parenting is a key determinant of a child's physical and mental health. Parenting, however, takes place in a social and economic context and is influenced by social norms and government policies in relation to families (Taylor et al, 2000). There is evidence that poor social circumstances impose particular stresses on parenting and reduce parents' ability to cope with the pressures and complexities of parenting (Ghate and Hazel, 2004).

## Trends in inequalities in health outcomes

Limited data are available on trends in health inequalities in pregnancy and early childhood in the UK, though the data that exist suggest that in most cases existing health inequalities are persisting or in some instances widening (see Chapter Three of this volume for further discussion of widening health inequalities). The gap in the infant mortality rate (IMR) between 'routine and manual' groups and the population as a whole, targeted to reduce by 10% by 2010, increased for the period 2001-03 compared with 1997-99 (see Table 5.1) (DH, 2005, p 27).

As the Department of Health status report acknowledges (DH, 2005, p 27), the trends shown in the table tend to mask the full extent of social differences in the IMR, as those in 'routine and manual' groups are not the most disadvantaged group and comparison is made with the whole population rather than the most privileged social group. The most disadvantaged infants are those born to single mothers and their IMR has decreased marginally from 7.6 per 1,000 live births in 1997-99 to 7.2 per 1,000 in 2001-03. The ratio of IMR among

**Table 5.1: Trends in three-year average infant mortality rates comparing National Statistics Socioeconomic Classification (NS SEC) routine and manual groups with all within marriage and joint registration births**

| | NS SEC90 | | | | NS SEC* | | | |
|---|---|---|---|---|---|---|---|---|
| | 1994-96 | 1995-97 | 1996-98 | 1997-99 | 1998-2000 | 1999-2001 | 2000-02 | 2001-03 |
| Infant deaths per 1,000 live births | | | | Baseline period | | | | |
| All within marriage and joint registrations | 5.9 | 5.8 | 5.7 | 5.6 | 5.4 | 5.3 | 5.2 | 5.0 |
| NS SEC three-class version – routine and manual group | 6.7 | 6.6 | 6.4 | 6.3 | 6.2 | 6.2 | 6.0 | 6.0 |
| Ratio: routine and manual/all | 1.15 | 1.14 | 1.12 | 1.13 | 1.14 | 1.17 | 1.16 | 1.19 |

*Notes:*
a) Figures for live births are a 10% sample coded for father's occupation.
b) Information on the father's occupation is not collected for births outside marriage if the father does not attend the baby's birth.
* Using NS SEC90 for data up to 2000 and NS SEC for 2001-03 data.
*Source:* ONS (2006)

infants of single mothers compared with all within marriage and joint registered births increased from 1.29 to 1.44 between 1997-99 and 2001-03.

Against a background of falling infant mortality rates, social differences in neonatal mortality rates appear to have reduced, but wide social differences persist in post-neonatal mortality (Maher and Macfarlane, 2004; Dummer and Parker, 2005). Inequalities in low birth-weight in Scotland narrowed in the early 1990s but increased again in the late 1990s (Fairley, 2005). Over the period 1983-2001, there was no evidence of change in social inequalities in cerebral palsy in the West Sussex region of the UK (Spencer – unpublished data). Between 1999 and 2004, there was no evidence of increasing prevalence of mental disorders in childhood and no change in the pattern of social inequalities (Green et al, 2004). Trends in childhood obesity suggest an emerging pattern of social inequality (Stamatakis et al, 2005).

## Trends in inequalities in health determinants

Trends in inequalities related to ethnicity/racism, housing, nutrition and smoking are discussed in other chapters in this book (see Chapters Six, Seven, Eight and Nine). Trends in income, poverty, employment, education and early childcare are discussed later in relation to New Labour's policy initiatives. Trends in family structure are less influenced by government policy, although fiscal policy and childcare policy can alleviate or exacerbate the inequalities associated with lone parenthood. The number of dependent children living in lone-parent households has more than tripled since 1972, although the proportion only increased very slightly from 22% to 23% between 2001 and 2005 (ONS, 2006).

## Life course impact of pregnancy and early childhood inequalities

Fetal life and the early years are key periods in the life course as, for some later outcomes, they are critical periods in which an exposure has an adverse or protective effect on development and subsequent disease outcome that is not significantly modified by subsequent exposure (Ben-Shlomo and Kuh, 2002). Exposures in pregnancy and early childhood may also act as the starting point of trajectories of risk that track into adult life and have an impact across the life course (Bartley et al, 1994; Power and Hertzman, 1999; Hertzman et al, 2001; Graham and Power, 2004). There are likely to be at least two elements to this process. First, adverse early life experiences lead to childhood ill health that persists into adulthood. Second, adverse early life circumstances continue into adulthood and are, in turn, associated with adult ill health (Graham and Power, 2004).

## Mechanisms by which pregnancy and early childhood inequalities develop

Although these early childhood health inequalities are widely recognised, the mechanisms by which they arise are less well understood. As has been observed in relation to many adult health outcomes, there is a finely graded stepwise increase in risk of many but not all adverse pregnancy and early childhood outcomes as social status decreases. Different explanations have been advanced to explain these social gradients in adulthood (see Chapter Four for a detailed discussion of the explanations for social gradients). In pregnancy and early childhood, it seems likely that gradients are the result of a number of possible processes: socially patterned risk and protective exposures that occur at critical periods in the life of the mother or the fetus (Barker, 1998) or that accumulate over time and operate across generations (Spencer, 2004; Kahn et al, 2005). In addition, socially patterned risk and protective exposures cluster in such a way that the more disadvantaged are exposed in pregnancy and early childhood to a high concentration of risk factors and the more privileged to a high concentration of protective factors. The relative importance of structure and agency in relation to these risk and protective exposures is the subject of debate, but many of the influences that underpin the exposures, such as nutrition, housing, employment and levels of social protection, are societal in origin and individuals have little control over them (see Chapters Four, Eight and Eleven for further discussion of structure and agency).

Cumulative intergenerational influences can be illustrated by the example of low birth-weight. Compared with a woman whose parents were advantaged, a woman whose parents were disadvantaged is more likely to have been of low birth-weight herself, to have experienced more childhood ill health, to have had a less nutritious diet with adverse effects on her growth leading to relative stunting and anaemia, to have started smoking in adolescence, to come to pregnancy at an earlier age and to smoke during pregnancy. These factors make it more likely that her babies will be born with low birth-weight. The more disadvantaged the woman, the more likely she is to have experienced increasing numbers of risk factors and fewer protective factors.

## Policy interventions

The foregoing discussion shows that inequalities in pregnancy and early childhood have a powerful impact on the health of mothers, infants and young children and these impacts may track into later childhood and adult life. The government has explicitly recognised this impact and set out policies to tackle health inequalities, endorsing the view of the Acheson Inquiry (Acheson, 1998) that strategies aimed at young children and present and future mothers have the best chance of reducing future inequalities in mental and physical health. This section summarises the policy interventions introduced by New Labour that affect young children and present and future mothers and assesses the evidence for their effectiveness.

Many of the numerous initiatives taken by the government would not be expected to show clear evidence of effectiveness in the short term and some, such as improving the quality of education for disadvantaged children, are unlikely to result in changes in health for many years. Furthermore, there are time lags between the formulation of policy, its implementation and the collection and analysis of data to assess policy impact. Evaluation of policy initiatives, therefore, is necessarily limited but the general direction of early impact can be identified.

### Every child matters

In 2003, Labour published a consultation paper, known in the UK as a Green Paper, entitled *Every child matters* (HM Government, 2003) alongside the government's response to the report into the death of Victoria Climbié, a young girl murdered by her aunt and her aunt's partner after a prolonged period of abuse. Similar initiatives have been taken in the other three UK nations, for example Children First in Wales. The Green Paper focused on four key themes:

* increasing the focus on supporting families and carers;
* ensuring intervention takes place before children reach crisis point and protecting children from 'falling through the net';
* addressing the problems of weak accountability and poor integration highlighted by the Climbié report;
* ensuring that people who work with children are valued, supported and trained.

Following the consultation on the Green Paper, the 2004 Children Act was passed and, in November 2004, the strategy for children and young people aged 0 to 19 years in England, *Every child matters: Change for children* (HM Government, 2004), was published. All government departments were actively involved in the strategy, representing a welcome cross-government approach to improving the lives of children and their families. The strategy is outcome-orientated and five outcomes were identified following a consultation with children and young people:

* be healthy;
* stay safe;
* enjoy and achieve;
* make a positive contribution;
* achieve economic well-being.

The strategy is being monitored against these outcomes using targets and key indicators. A further organisational element of the strategy is the development of Children's Trusts.[1] These are designed to bring together all services for children and young people in an area, based on the 2004 Children Act duty to cooperate to focus on improving outcomes for all children and young people. Trusts will be expected to institute integrated strategies based on joint needs assessment, shared decisions on priorities, identification of all available resources, and joint plans to deploy them. Children's Trusts were piloted in 35 areas to test these integrated strategies.

The success of this broad programme will depend on the achievement of the outcomes outlined above. The government claims that its policies have had a positive impact on the health of children through a reduction in child traffic casualties and an increase in breastfeeding among low-income mothers but acknowledges that mental health problems and childhood obesity are on the increase (SEU, 2004).

As indicated above, there is limited evidence of trends in inequalities in pregnancy and early childhood health outcomes but what evidence is available suggests a persistence in the social differentials in infant mortality, an increase in inequality in birth-weight and an emerging social gradient in obesity.

There are limited data against which to measure the impact of recent child protection strategies, including Children's Trusts, and their contribution to staying safe. Child maltreatment deaths fell in the UK between the 1970s and mid-1990s (UNICEF, 2003). Child homicides, based on criminal statistics for England and Wales, showed a tendency towards increasing deaths between 1993 and 2003 in children under one year of age but not in other age groups, although the rates showed some wide fluctuations during the 10-year period.[2] Trends in child protection registration data are difficult to interpret because of changes in registration criteria. Despite fluctuations in registration for various categories of abuse and neglect, there is no evidence of a significant increase or decrease in the overall numbers registered in England between 1993 and 2003.[3] Of the four nations of the UK, Northern Ireland has the highest rate of registration and Scotland the lowest.

An initial evaluation of eight of the 35 pathfinder Children's Trusts, established in April 2004, reported positive progress in establishing innovative integrated services but the short period over which the Trusts had been operative precluded any evaluation of outcomes (NCB, 2005).

## Fiscal policy, child poverty reduction and social inclusion

There can be no doubt that the Labour government has taken poverty and social exclusion very seriously (Hills and Stewart, 2005). Its commitment to reducing child poverty has been addressed through both tax and benefit policies, such as increasing the level of child benefit and working families tax credits. Other planks of the child poverty reduction strategy have included increased education and training, and employment policy.

In 1997, soon after its election, the government established the Social Exclusion Unit (SEU) as an information resource to support cross-government policies to improve the life chances of the most disadvantaged groups in society. In June 2006, Hilary Armstrong was appointed as the first Social Exclusion Minister with a seat in the Cabinet. Much of the work of the SEU has focused on children and young people.

A key element of the strategy to reduce social exclusion with particular relevance to pregnancy and early childhood has been the focus on reducing teenage pregnancies, with a particular emphasis on pregnancies among girls below 18 years of age. The UK had one of the highest levels of teenage pregnancies in rich nations in the late 1990s (UNICEF, 2001). In one of its first reports, the SEU set out policy options for reducing teenage pregnancies (SEU, 1999). The report identified low expectations, ignorance and mixed messages from society related to teenage sexuality as three main factors underlying the UK's high teenage pregnancy rates. The SEU identified two main goals: reducing teenage conceptions with the specific aim of halving the rate of conceptions among those under 18 years of age by 2010; and getting more teenage parents into education, training or employment to reduce the risk of long-term social exclusion.

Maternity benefits, available to pregnant women who are not in receipt of statutory maternity pay, have been increased by New Labour by up to 50% in real terms to £108.85 per week, eligibility has been widened, and they are now paid for 26 rather than 18 weeks. Other benefits, such as income support or jobseeker's allowance, may be reduced or stopped while maternity allowance is being paid. In addition, the government has introduced a Sure Start maternity grant worth £500 for those on low income.

Recent legislation has increased parental leave entitlement. Ordinary maternity leave is 26 weeks independent of length of employment. Additional maternity leave is available for those who have worked for the same employer for 26 weeks by the end of the 15th week of pregnancy. Paternity leave has recently been introduced and is available to those men in work who have been working for the same employer for 26 weeks by the end of the 15th week of their partner's pregnancy, and are earning above the lower earning level for national insurance contributions. The entitlement is two weeks, which must be taken all together and within 56 days of the baby's birth. Since 1997, there is some evidence of redistribution of income in favour of the poor through government fiscal policy, although income inequality may have increased (Sutherland et al, 2003; Hills, 2004).

Tax and benefit reforms have resulted in higher child benefit and in the child tax credit that is of equal value to families out of work and to those in low-paid work (Hills, 2004). Child poverty in the UK, as measured by children in households with incomes less than 60% of national median income, fell from 34% in 1996/97 to 28% in 2002/03 (after housing costs) (Hills and Stewart, 2005, p 327). The UK, along with the US and Norway, is one of the few rich nations to show a reduction in child poverty in recent years (UNICEF, 2005). However, as the UNICEF publication indicates, child poverty rates are unlikely to fall below 10% unless at least 10% of gross domestic product (GDP) is devoted to social transfers. The 1999 UK level of social transfers was 7% (UNICEF, 2005). Findings from the Families and Children Study funded by the Department for Work and Pensions confirm the improvement for families with children showing a fall in the percentage of families experiencing financial hardship between 1999 and 2001 (Vegeris and Perry, 2003). Hills and Stewart (2005) caution that further reductions in child poverty rates will require more aggressive redistribution policies in coming years. Hirsch (2006) argues that it will cost around £30 billion between 2006 and 2020 to reduce child poverty to 5%. This is about 2% of GDP but less than one year's economic growth over the 14-year period. Achieving the target of eliminating child poverty by 2020 will require substantially higher taxation.

The teenage pregnancy rate has been in slow decline since 1999, but it is doubtful if government targets will be met (Bradshaw, 2006). However, Bradshaw (2006) points out that even if targets are reached, the impact on child poverty rates will be marginal as children of teenage mothers are a small proportion of the total in poverty.

UK maternity benefit and parental leave entitlements remain among the lowest in Europe despite the recent improvements. The Daycare Trust predicts that very few fathers will be able to take up the paternity leave entitlement because of the very low level of pay associated with Additional Paternity Leave.[4]

## Work and worklessness

Work, as a way out of poverty and a means of reducing child poverty in particular, has been a central theme of New Labour policy since 1997. Measures have been introduced to reduce youth unemployment (New Deal programmes), to encourage lone parents into work, and to reduce long-term unemployment.

Registered unemployment fell to a 30-year low in 2004 but has shown a slow increase since. The growth in the economy and government policies has succeeded in reducing long-term employment and increasing employment among lone parents (Hills and Stewart, 2005, p 331). The fall in unemployment and the increased number of families with children with someone in the workforce has been a major factor in reducing child poverty (Sutherland et al, 2003). The introduction of a minimum wage has also contributed to reducing working poverty, although wage levels for unskilled workers remain among the lowest in Europe (UNICEF, 2001; see also Chapter Eight in this volume). However, economic inactivity rates have only fallen slowly for women and have risen for men (Hills and Stewart, 2005, p 331). The impact of the New Deal has been limited and unemployment rates among 16- to 17-year-olds remain unchanged. By European standards, the UK has a high level of households with children in which no adult is working, despite falling from 20% in 1996 (UNICEF, 2001) to 17.6% in 2003/04 (DWP, 2005). The high proportion of children in workless households along with the high percentage of full-time workers with earnings less than two thirds of the average wage is likely to account for the high level of child poverty in the UK compared with other European countries (UNICEF, 2001; Hirsch, 2006).

## Public health policies

The public health White Paper, *Choosing health* (DH, 2004a), is the centrepiece of the government's public health policy for England. One of its main aims is to reduce health inequalities. As suggested in Chapter Four of this volume, the White Paper is informed by theories of individual behaviour and choice as the drivers of health and health inequalities. The section in the White Paper on children and young people recognises the need to reduce child health inequalities and highlights child poverty reduction as a major component of this strategy. However, the section of the White Paper referred to above lays most emphasis on service reorganisation and on promoting healthy lifestyles as the means to reduce child health inequalities (DH, 2004, pp 40-76). The Child Health Promotion programme, set out in the *National service framework for children, young people and maternity services* (DH, 2004b), is presented as a 'joined up system to ensure health and wellbeing for children and young people from birth to adulthood' (DH, 2004b, p 44). It is specifically viewed as a broad-based programme of support to children and their families as a means of addressing the wider determinants of health and health inequalities. Its key components are assessment of the child's and family's needs, health promotion, childhood screening, immunisations, early interventions to address identified needs, and safeguarding children from harm.

The White Paper characterises lifestyle factors such as smoking and poor diet that contribute to child health inequalities as resulting from unhealthy choices. Health inequalities are explicitly seen as arising from 'the cumulative results of thousands of choices by millions of people that impact on health' (DH, 2004a, p 15). Consistent with this explanation of health inequalities, the White Paper sets out to reduce inequalities through making healthier choices easier for children and their families and providing information and support in pregnancy and in the early years of a child's life.

Evaluation of the impact of *Choosing health* is unrealistic this early after its publication. However, on theoretical grounds, as suggested in Chapters Three and Four of this volume, there is good reason to believe that the choice agenda, on which it is based, will increase rather than decrease health inequalities. There are three major reasons for this: first, health is not chosen but moulded and shaped by social and environmental circumstances interacting with biological factors; second, the lifestyle choices to which the document refers are more easily made by those with greater social power, status and assets; and third, health inequalities are only partially explained by lifestyle factors. In addition, much activity in the *Choosing health* action plans is channelled through services focused on older children.

## Sure Start, Children's Centres and early childcare

Sure Start, based on carefully researched US projects, is the major recent government initiative related to early childhood. It is targeted at young children and their families in disadvantaged areas and is intended to produce examples of good practice that can be 'mainstreamed' in the future. Areas had to bid for funding and demonstrate local need and involvement of local communities. The first wave of 60 Sure Start programmes had funding approved in June 2000. There have been five further waves resulting in a total of 522 local programmes by 2004. These programmes target 400,000 children aged 0-4 years in the most deprived 20% of areas of England. Each programme has roughly £1,000 to spend on each child over the seven- to 10-year period of the programme's expected lifetime. All the programmes are locally designed but are expected to achieve nationally set targets. The programmes can have different emphases but common features are outreach and home visiting, parenting support, support for good-quality play, learning and childcare experience, primary healthcare and advice, and support for parents and children with special needs.

The ring-fenced resources to support Sure Start programmes are being phased out with the strategic aim of incorporating innovative Sure Start services into mainstream services through Children's Centres. The government is committed to establishing a Sure Start Children's Centre in every community by 2010 so that every family will have access to an affordable, flexible, high-quality childcare place for their child. It is envisaged that these centres will provide integrated education, care, family support and health services. In 2004, the government published a 10-year strategy for childcare (HM Treasury, 2004) that incorporated Children's Centres as a key component. The strategy aims to provide choice and flexibility; availability, with a target of 15 hours a week for 38 weeks of free, high-quality childcare by 2010 and 20 hours a week by 2014; quality, with improved career structure for childcare workers and strengthened inspection and regulation; and affordability, with an increase in the limits of the childcare element of the working tax credit. The 2006 Childcare Act is now being implemented as part of this strategy.

Sure Start was also established in Wales, Scotland and Northern Ireland, but under the direction of the devolved administrations. Sure Start Wales was incorporated into the Children and Youth Support Fund

(Cymorth) in 2003 that is administered through Children and Young People's Partnerships within each local authority. Cymorth covers ages 0-25 and each local authority has been asked to establish at least one integrated Children's Centre bringing together all local statutory agencies. In Scotland, Sure Start funding remains ring-fenced and the Scottish Executive has allocated funds to all 32 local authorities with guaranteed funding beyond 2008.

Sure Start has introduced innovative initiatives in many areas, although their effectiveness has been difficult to measure. Despite relatively high levels of expenditure, only a small percentage of disadvantaged children have access to the programme and the early results of national evaluation are disappointing (Belsky et al, 2006) in showing little immediate impact, though much of the benefit of such schemes is likely to be in the medium to long term. Targeting the programmes to the most deprived 20% of areas of the country has resulted in many poor children having no access to the programmes and even in the areas covered by the programmes many families have failed to access the services. The evidence so far from the national evaluation suggests that the most deprived children are least likely to benefit from Sure Start (Belsky et al, 2006).

Children's Trusts and Children's Centres are being piloted in some areas, but results are as yet limited. The Change for Children agenda in England shows promising attention to children's issues, but is yet to be fully implemented and tested in practice. The intention is to mainstream some of the initiatives pioneered by Sure Start programmes as part of this agenda. The concern is that the additional funds needed to support these developments may not be forthcoming. Norman Glass, the man credited with promoting Sure Start within the Treasury, was quoted as saying:

> Something had to give if there were to be 3,500 Children's Centres, if they were to be funded on the same basis as the local Sure Starts and were to expand at the required rate and rolled out in tandem with a general raising of childcare standards. ... What gave was the autonomy of the 'local' Sure Starts and their 'generous' funding. The programmes are to be wound up within the next two years and folded back into local government control. No more management boards with local parents and volunteers, a severe cut in funding per head so it can be spread over 3,500 Children's Centres: and no more ring fencing. (Glass, 2005)

Despite the introduction by the government of a National Childcare Strategy in 1998, progress towards targets has been slow (Skinner, 2006). By 2005, a total of 582,000 new childcare and early education places had been created, but provision remains patchy, and there are insufficient places for disabled children, for children from ethnic minorities, and disadvantaged children (Skinner, 2006). Sure Start and other initiatives related to early childcare have not yet succeeded in narrowing the gap between childcare provision in the UK and much of the rest of Europe. Many families continue to be excluded from early childcare by high costs inhibiting the movement of lone parents off benefits and into work (Daycare Trust, 2004), and going to work is associated with reduced duration of breastfeeding, especially if full-time and if return to work is soon after birth (Hawkins et al, 2007).

## Education and health policies

Education and health policies form an important part of social protection and poor families stand to benefit most from higher levels of public spending on these policy areas. Parental education plays a key role in the early years, affecting parents' interest in their children's education, influencing the child's motivation and aspirations, and affecting child development (McKnight et al, 2005). Spending on both education and health services has increased significantly under New Labour, with the annual growth rate of education expenditure increasing from 1.2% between 1996-97 and 1999-2000 to a planned 7.4% between 2002-03 and 2005-06 and that of health expenditure from 3.2% to a planned 7.6% in the same time periods (Hills, 2004, p 218). Extensive service reforms have accompanied increased spending in both sectors.

As improved education and healthcare are long-term strategies for reduction in health inequalities and child poverty, it is difficult to judge the effects of increased levels of education and health expenditure and the government's reform programmes at this time. However, in order to reverse the decline in social mobility and the continued close link between parental income and a child's educational achievement, future education policy will have to tip the balance of education very much in favour of low-income children. It will also be important to ensure that the introduction of market reforms within the NHS does not jeopardise access to and affordability of healthcare by poor children and their families.

## What further needs to be done?

In sharp contrast to previous UK governments, the current administration has made women and children a key focus of policy. It has committed considerable resources to this policy agenda. However, as noted earlier, there remains much to do if inequalities in pregnancy and early life are to be effectively challenged and reduced. The following bullet points summarise the broad areas of policy necessary:

- further reduction of child poverty – a need to increase benefits and the minimum wage, probably by increasing social transfers;
- further improvement of parental leave provision to the best European levels;
- further reduction in unwanted pregnancies, particularly in young and vulnerable women;
- improvement of maternal health, in particular promoting nutrition and reducing smoking and substance misuse;
- provision of affordable childcare for all parents including those on low (or no) incomes and promotion of family-friendly working practices and employment;
- provision of universal high-quality services such as those being developed through Sure Start, with targeting of increased resources to disadvantaged areas;
- simplification of child and family service provision by organisational change such as that proposed in *Every child matters*.

These changes should be underpinned by:

- adequate, sustained and dedicated financial and other resources;
- international comparative research, with the aim of identifying key welfare, social and fiscal policies associated with better child health and well-being and reduction of inequalities;
- further research on the mechanisms by which social circumstances influence health and well-being across the life course;
- rigorous evaluation of policy.

### Notes

[1] www.everychildmatters.gov.uk/aims/childrenstrusts, accessed 26 June 2006.

[2] 'Child Protection Statistics: 5. Child deaths', www.nspcc.org.uk/inform, accessed 27 June 2006.

[3] 'Child Protection Statistics: 2. Child protection in the family', www.nspcc.org.uk/inform, accessed 27 June 2006.

[4] www.daycaretrust.org.uk/mod/fileman/DTI_Paternity_May06.pdf, accessed 25 August 2006.

## References

Acheson, D. (1998) *Independent inquiry into inequalities in health*, London: The Stationery Office.

Adelman, L., Middleton, S. and Ashworth, K. (2003) *Britain's poorest children: Severe and persistent poverty and social exclusion*, London: Save the Children.

Baldwin, N. and Spencer, N.J. (1999) 'Strategic planning to prevent harm to children', in N. Baldwin (ed) *Protecting children: Promoting their rights? A reader in theory and practice*, London: Whiting and Birch.

Bambang, S., Spencer, N.J., Logan, S. and Gill, L. (2000) 'Cause-specific perinatal death rates, birth weight and deprivation in the West Midlands, 1991-93', *Child: Care, Health and Development*, vol 26, no 1, pp 73-82.

Barker, D.J.P. (1998) *Mothers, babies and health in later life*, Edinburgh: Churchill Livingston.

Bartley, M., Power, C., Blane, D., Davey Smith, G. and Shipley, M. (1994) 'Birth weight and later socioeconomic disadvantage: evidence from the 1958 British cohort study', *BMJ*, vol 309, pp 1475-9.

Belsky, J., Melhuish, E., Barnes, J., Leyland, A.H. and Romaniuk, H. (2006) 'Effects of local Sure Start programmes on children and families: early findings from a quasi-experimental, cross-sectional study', *BMJ*, vol 332, pp 1476-83.

Ben-Shlomo, Y. and Kuh, D. (2002) 'A lifecourse approach to chronic disease epidemiology: conceptual models, empirical challenges, and interdisciplinary perspectives', *International Journal of Epidemiology*, vol 31, no 2, pp 285-93.

Blackburn, C., Spencer, N., Bonas, S., Coe, C., Dolan, A. and Moy, R. (2003) 'Effect of strategies to reduce exposure of infants to environmental tobacco smoke in the home: cross sectional survey', *BMJ*, vol 327, pp 257-62.

Blair, T. (1999) 'Beveridge revisited: a welfare state for the 21st century', in R. Walker (ed) *Ending child poverty: Popular welfare for the 21st century*, Bristol: The Policy Press.

Bradshaw, J. (2006) *Teenage births*, York: Joseph Rowntree Foundation.

Caldwell, J. (1979) 'Education as a factor in mortality decline: an examination of Nigerian data', *Population Studies*, vol 33, pp 395-413.

Cawson, P., Wattam, C., Brooker, S. and Kelly, G. (2000) *Child maltreatment in the United Kingdom: A study of the prevalence of child abuse and neglect*, London: National Society for the Prevention of Cruelty to Children.

CEMACH (Confidential Enquiry into Maternal and Child Health) (2004) *Why mothers die*, London: CEMACH.

Chevalier, A., Harmon, C., O'Sullivan, V. and Walker, I. (2005) *Impact of parental income and education on schooling of their children*, London: Institute for Fiscal Studies.

Daycare Trust (2004) *A new era for universal child care?*, London: Daycare Trust.

DH (Department of Health) (2003) *Tackling health inequalities: A Programme for Action*, London: DH.

DH (2004a) *Choosing health: Making healthier choices easier*, Cm 6374, London: The Stationery Office.

DH (2004b) *National service framework for children, young people and maternity services* (www.dh.gov.uk/PolicyandGuidance/HealthandSocialCareTopics/ChildrensServices/ChildServicesInformation/ChildServicesInformationArticle/fs/en?CONTENT_ID=4089111&chk=U8Ecln, accessed 6 June 2006).

DH (2005) *Tackling health inequalities: Status report on the Programme for Action*, London: DH.

Dolk, H., Pattenden, S. and Johnson, A. (2001) 'Cerebral palsy, low birthweight and socio-economic deprivation: inequalities in a major cause of childhood disability', *Paediatric and Perinatal Epidemiology*, vol 15, no 4, pp 359-63.

Dowding, V.M. and Barry, C. (1990) 'Cerebral palsy: social class differences in prevalence in relation to birth weight and severity of disability', *Journal of Epidemiology and Community Health*, vol 44, no 3, pp 191-5.

Drever, F. and Whitehead, M. (1997) *Health inequalities: Decennial Supplement (DS No 15)*, London: The Stationery Office.

Dummer, T.J.B. and Parker, L. (2005) 'Changing socioeconomic inequality in infant mortality in Cumbria', *Archives of Disease in Childhood*, vol 90, no 2, pp 157-62.

—

Dummer, T.J.B., Dickinson, H.O., Pearce, M.S., Charlton, M.E. and Parker, L. (2000) 'Stillbirth risk with social class and deprivation: no evidence for increasing inequalities', *Journal of Clinical Epidemiology*, vol 53, no 2, pp 147-55.

DWP (Department for Work and Pensions) (2005) *Households below average income, 2003/4*, London: DWP.

Fairley, L. (2005) 'Changing patterns of inequality in birthweight and its determinants: a population-based study, Scotland 1980-2000', *Paediatric and Perinatal Epidemiology*, vol 19, no 5, pp 342-51.

Fairley, L. and Leyland, A.H. (2006) 'Social inequalities in perinatal outcomes: Scotland 1980-2000', *Journal of Epidemiology and Community Health*, vol 60, no 1, pp 31-6.

Ferguson, S.E., Smith, G.N., Salenieks, M.E., Windrim, R. and Walker, M.C. (2002) 'Preterm premature rupture of membranes: nutritional and socioeconomic factors', *Journal of Obstetrics and Gynaecology*, vol 100, no 6, pp 1250-6.

Ghate, D. and Hazel, N. (2004) *Parenting in poor environments: Stress, support, and coping*, London: Policy Research Bureau.

Glass, N. (2005) 'Surely some mistake?', *The Guardian*, 5 January.

Graham, H. and Power, C. (2004) *Childhood disadvantage and adult health: A lifecourse framework*, London: Health Development Agency.

Green, H., McGinnity, A., Meltzer, H., Ford, T. and Goodman, R. (2004) *Mental health of children and young people 2004*, London: Palgrave Macmillan.

Gudmundsson, S., Bjorgvinsdottir, L., Molin, J., Gunnarsson, G. and Marsal, K. (1997) 'Socioeconomic status and perinatal outcome according to residence area in the city of Malmo', *Acta Obstetrica Gynaecologica Scandinavica*, vol 76, no 4, pp 318-23.

Hawkins, S.S., Griffiths, L.J., Dezateux, C., Law, C. and the Millennium Cohort Study Child Health Group (2007) 'Maternal employment and breast-feeding initiation: findings from the Millennium Cohort Study', *Paediatric and Perinatal Epidemiology*, vol 21, no 13, pp 242-7.

Hemminki, K., Niemi, M.L., Saloniemi, I., Vainio, H. and Hemminki, E. (1980) 'Spontaneous abortions by occupation and social class in Finland', *International Journal of Epidemiology*, vol 9, no 2, pp 149-53.

Hertzman, C., Power, C., Matthews, S. and Manor, O. (2001) 'Using an interactive framework of society and lifecourse to explain self-rated health in early adulthood', *Social Science and Medicine*, vol 53, no 12, pp 1575-85.

Hills, J. (2004) *Inequality and the state*, Oxford: Oxford University Press.

Hills, J. and Stewart, K. (2005) *A more equal society? New Labour, poverty, inequality and exclusion*, Bristol: The Policy Press.

Hirsch, D. (2006) *What will it take to end child poverty? Firing on all cylinders*, York: Joseph Rowntree Foundation.

HM Government (2003) *Every child matters*, Cm 5860, London: HMSO.

HM Government (2004) *Every child matters: Change for children*, London: HMSO.

HM Treasury (2004) *Choice for parents, the best start for children: A ten year strategy for childcare*, London: HMSO.

James, W.P.T., Nelson, M., Ralph, A. and Leather, S. (1997) 'Socioeconomic determinants of health: the contribution of nutrition to inequalities in health', *BMJ*, vol 314, pp 1545-8.

Jefferis, B.J.H.M., Power, C. and Hertzman, C. (2002) 'Birthweight, childhood socioeconomic environment, and cognitive development in the 1958 British birth cohort study, *BMJ*, vol 325, pp 305-11.

Kahn, R.S., Wilson, K. and Wise, P.H. (2005) 'Intergenerational health disparities: socioeconomic status, women's health conditions, and children's behaviour'. *Public Health Reports*, vol 120, no 4, pp 399-408.

Kendrick, D. and Marsh, P. (2001) 'How useful are sociodemographic characteristics in identifying children at risk of unintentional injury?', *Public Health*, vol 115, no 2, pp 103-7.

Kramer, M.S., Séguin, L., Lydon, J. and Goulet, L. (2000) 'Socio-economic disparities in pregnancy outcome: why do the poor fare so poorly?', *Paediatric and Perinatal Epidemiology*, vol 14, no 3, pp 194-210.

Laflamme, L. and Diderichsen, F. (2000) 'Social differences in traffic injury risks in childhood and youth – a literature review and research agenda', *Injury Prevention*, vol 6, no 4, pp 293-8.

Li, J. and Taylor, B. (1993) 'Factors affecting uptake of measles, mumps, rubella immunisation' *BMJ*, vol 307, pp 168-71.

Maher, J. and Macfarlane, A. (2004) 'Inequalities in infant mortality: trends by social class, registration status, mother's age and birthweight, England and Wales, 1976-2000', *Health Statistics Quarterly*, Winter, vol 24, pp 14-22.

Manning, D., Brewster, B. and Bundred, P. (2005) 'Social deprivation and admission for neonatal care', *Archives of Disease in Childhood Fetal and Neonatal Edition*, vol 90, no 4, pp F337-8.

McKnight, A, Gennester, H. and Lupton, R. (2005) 'Education, education, education …: an assessment of Labour's success in tackling education inequalities', in J. Hills and K. Stewart (eds) *A more equal society? New Labour, poverty, inequality and exclusion*, Bristol:The Policy Press, pp 47-68.

Meltzer, H., Gatwood, R., Goodman, R. and Ford, T. (2000) *The mental health of children and adolescents in Great Britain*, London:The Stationery Office.

NCB (National Children's Bureau) (2005) *Realising children's trust arrangements: National evaluation of children's trusts, Phase 1 report*, London: NCB with the University of East Anglia.

ONS (Office of National Statistics) (2006) *Social Trends No. 36, 2006 edition*, London: Palgrave Macmillan.

Pallotto, E.K. and Kilbride, H.W. (2006) 'Perinatal outcome and later implications of intra-uterine growth restriction', *Clinical Obstetrics and Gynaecology*, vol 49, no 2, pp 257-69.

Papadimitriou, G., Kotzaeridou, U., Mouratidis, C., Goularas, P., Coe, C., Ganas, A. and Spencer, N. (2005) 'Rates and social patterning of household smoking and breastfeeding in contrasting European settings', *Child: Care, Health and Development*, vol 31, no 5, pp 603-10.

Pharoah, P.O., Stephenson, C.J., Cook, R.W. and Stephenson, R.C. (1994) 'Clinical and sub-clinical deficits at 8 years in a geographically defined cohort of low birthweight infants', *Archives of Disease in Childhood*, vol 70, no 4, pp 264-70.

Ponce, N.A., Hoggatt, K.J., Wilhelm, M. and Ritz, B. (2005) 'Preterm birth: the interaction of traffic-related air pollution with economic hardship in Los Angeles neighborhoods', *American Journal of Epidemiology*, vol 162, no 2, pp 140-8.

Power, C. and Hertzman, C. (1999) 'Health, well-being, and coping skills', in D.P. Keating and C. Hertzman (eds) *Developmental health and the wealth of nations: Social, biological and educational dynamics*, New York, NY, and London: Guilford Press.

Quigley, M.A., Cumberland, P., Cowden, J.M. and Rodrigues, L.C. (2006) 'How protective is breastfeeding against diarrhoeal disease in infants in 1990s England? A case-control study', *Archives of Disease in Childhood*, vol 91, no 3, pp 245-50.

Relton, C.L., Pearce, M.S. and Parker, L. (2005) 'The influence of erythrocyte folate and serum vitamin B12 status on birth weight', *British Journal of Nutrition*, vol 93, no 5, pp 593-9.

Samad, L., Tate, A., Dezateux, C., Peckham, C., Butler, N. and Bedford, H. (2006) 'Differences in risk factors for partial and no immunisation in the first year of life', *BMJ*, vol 332, pp 1312-13.

Séguin, L., Xu, Q., Gauvin, L., Zunzunegui, M.V., Potvin, L. and Frohlich, K.L. (2005) 'Undertanding the dimension of socioeconomic status that influence toddlers' health: unique impact of lack of money for basic needs in Quebec's birth cohort', *Journal of Epidemiology and Community Health*, vol 59, no 1, pp 42-8.

SEU (Social Exclusion Unit) (1999) *Teenage pregnancy*, London: HMSO.

SEU (2004) *Breaking the cycle: Taking stock of progress and priorities for the future*, London: HMSO.

Sidebotham, P. and Heron, J., and the ALSPAC Study Team (2006) 'Child maltreatment in the "Children of the Nineties": a cohort study of risk factors', *Child Abuse & Neglect*, vol 30, no 5, pp 497-522.

Skinner, C. (2006) *How can childcare help to end child poverty?*, York: Joseph Rowntree Foundation.

Spencer, N. (2003) *Weighing the evidence: How is birthweight determined?*, Abingdon: Radcliffe Press.

Spencer, N.J. (2004) 'Accounting for the social disparity in birthweight: results from an intergenerational study', *Journal of Epidemiology and Community Health*, vol 58, no 5, pp 418-19.

Spencer, N.J. (2005) 'Does material disadvantage explain the increased risk of adverse health, educational and behavioural outcomes among children in lone parent households in Britain? A cross-sectional study', *Journal of Epidemiology and Community Health*, vol 59, no 2, pp 152-7.

Spencer, N. and Coe, C. (2003a) 'Parent reported longstanding health problems in early childhood: a cohort study', *Archives of Disease in Childhood*, vol 88, no 7, pp 570-3.

Spencer, N. and Coe, C. (2003b) 'Social patterning and prediction of parent-reported behaviour problems at 3 years in a cohort study', *Child: Care, Health and Development*, vol 29, no 5, pp 329-36.

Stamatakis, E., Primatesta, P., Chinn, S., Rona, R. and Falacheti, E. (2005) 'Overweight and obesity trends from 1974 to 2001 in English children: what is the role of socioeconomic status?', *Archives of Disease in Childhood*, vol 90, no 10, pp 999-1004.

Sundrum, R., Logan, S., Wallace, A. and Spencer, N.J. (2005) 'Cerebral plasy and socio-economic status: a retrospective cohort study', *Archives of Disease in Childhood*, vol 90, no 1, pp 15-18.

Sutherland, H., Sefton, T. and Piachaud, D. (2003) *Poverty in Britain: The impact of government policy since 1997*, London: Joseph Rowntree Foundation.

Taylor, J., Spencer, N.J. and Baldwin, N. (2000) 'The social, economic and political context of parenting', *Archives of Disease in Childhood*, vol 82, no 2, pp 113-20.

UNICEF (2001) *A league table of teenage births in rich nations. Innocenti report card no.3*, Florence: UNICEF Innocenti Research Centre.

UNICEF (2003) *A league table of child maltreatment in rich nations. Innocenti report card no.5*, Florence: UNICEF Innocenti Research Centre.

UNICEF (2005) *A league table of child poverty in rich nations. Innocenti research report*, Florence: UNICEF Innocenti Research Centre.

Vegeris, S. and Perry, J. (2003) *Families and children 2001: Living standards and the children: Research Report 190*, London: Department for Work and Pensions.

Webber, R. and Butler, T. (2006) *Classifying pupils by where they live: How well does this predict variations in their GCSE results? CASA Working Paper 99*, London: Centre for Advanced Spatial Analysis, University College London.

Woodroffe C., Glickman M., Barker, M. and Power, C. (1993) *Children, teenagers and health: The key data*, Milton Keynes: Open University Press.

Wright, J. and Polack, C. (2006) 'Understanding variation in measles-mumps-rubella immunization coverage – a population-based study', *European Journal of Public Health*, vol 16, no 2, pp 137-42.

# SIX

# Inequalities and ethnicity: evidence and intervention

*Hannah Bradby and Tarani Chandola*

## Introduction

The Acheson Report (Acheson, 1998) included a chapter on 'Ethnicity', an important dimension of inequalities in health in the UK. The chapter acknowledged the difficulties in defining ethnicity and considered evidence on health inequalities from different definitions of ethnicity. Apart from documenting the patterns of morbidity and mortality among the major ethnic groups living in Britain, the report noted differences in socioeconomic status between ethnic groups. Unemployment, poverty and poor housing conditions among Pakistani and Bangladeshi households were highlighted as potentially contributing to their poorer health in general. However, there remains considerable debate about specific factors that underlie both ethnic differences in health and differences in health within ethnic groups.

The inquiry made recommendations in two general areas: first, general policies targeted at disadvantaged socioeconomic groups in which minority ethnic groups are disproportionately represented; and second, policies specifically targeted at ameliorating health service access for minority ethnic groups. As minority ethnic communities typically contain a higher proportion of households with children, living in disadvantaged socioeconomic conditions, these communities should benefit from general policies targeted at mothers, children and families and those related to education, employment, poverty and housing. The inquiry argued that separate policies for minority ethnic groups risked marginalising minority ethnic issues, with the implication that the health problems in minority ethnic groups are different from those in the ethnic majority, with different causes and different solutions. Any such implication would run counter to the evidence that suggests that the similarities between ethnic groups in the causes of health inequalities are greater than the differences (Bhopal, 1997).

On the other hand, the inquiry also acknowledged that failure to consider minority ethnic issues risked increasing ethnic inequalities by unintentionally favouring policies that benefited the ethnic majority. So the inquiry also made recommendations specific to ethnic minorities. These were:

- the further development of services that are sensitive to the needs of minority ethnic people and that promote greater awareness of their health risks; and
- the specific consideration of minority ethnic groups in needs assessment, resource allocation, healthcare planning and provision.

In addition, as data on the health of minority ethnic groups are particularly hard to collect and are based on inappropriate definitions of ethnicity, the inquiry's general recommendation to improve the capacity to monitor inequalities in health and their determinants is especially valid for ethnic minorities.

This chapter will update the evidence available on health patterns among ethnic groups by considering significant findings from data sets that have become available since the report of the Acheson Inquiry was published. The Acheson Report examined evidence on the major ethnic groups and so 'excluded' other minority groups such as religious and cultural groups and the Traveller/Roma communities. In addition to new findings from new data sets, this chapter considers some evidence on access to and use of health services by ethnic groups and how the responsibilities of public services have changed with the 1999 publication of Sir William Macpherson's report on the Stephen Lawrence inquiry and the Race Relations (Amendment) Act in 2000. Finally, we return to the dilemma of general and specific policies and their likely effects on health inequalities. In conclusion, recommendations for tackling inequalities are made.

## Post-Acheson Report evidence on health patterns

### New data

Since the Acheson Report's publication, four significant population representative sources of data have become available that add to the overall picture. The first of these is the 2001 census variables on ethnicity. In the England and Wales 2001 census, Pakistani and Bangladeshi men and women in England and Wales reported the highest rates of 'not good' health in 2001 (ONS, 2005). Pakistanis had age-standardised rates of 'not good' health of 13% (men) and 17% (women). The age-standardised rates for Bangladeshis were 14% (men) and 15% (women).

These rates, which take account of the difference in age structures between the ethnic groups, were around twice those of their White British counterparts. Chinese men and women were the least likely to report their health as 'not good'.

Second, the ethnicity data in the ONS Longitudinal Study have been used to describe patterns of morbidity and mortality (Harding and Rosato, 1999; Harding and Balarajan, 2000; Harding and Balarajan, 2001) as well as test complex hypotheses about intergenerational changes in the associations about ethnicity and health. For example, for South Asians and Black Caribbeans poor health has persisted across generations, and for Black Africans health has worsened (Harding and Balarajan, 2000). Among mothers of Black Caribbean, Black African, Indian, Pakistani and Bangladeshi ethnicity, mean birth-weights of infants of migrant mothers were similar to those of infants whose mothers were born in the UK, contrary to the expectation that UK-born minority ethnic mothers would have higher birth-weight babies than migrant mothers (Harding et al, 2004). In terms of social mobility, between 1971 and 1981 there was some upward social mobility among South Asian and West Indian migrants, but most minority ethnic groups remained socially stable, and relatively disadvantaged compared with the majority population (Harding and Balarajan, 2001). Social disadvantage persists across generations of ethnic minorities. Evidence from the life-course literature shows that the accumulation of disadvantage across the life course results in poorer health trajectories. This suggests that an increase in health inequalities among ethnic minorities and migrants can be expected (Harding and Balarajan, 2001).

Third, the EMPIRIC (Ethnic Minority Psychiatric Illness Rates in the Community) study (Sproston and Nazroo, 2002), a quantitative and qualitative survey of rates of mental illness among different ethnic groups in England, published its findings. This study showed that Black Caribbean people do not have significantly higher prevalence of psychotic illnesses compared to the White majority group, whereas they do show much higher rates of first contact with treatment services for such illnesses. In contrast to studies on rates of contact with services, the EMPIRIC study indicated a twofold higher rate for Black Caribbean people compared with the White group. This difference was not significant for men or the total Black Caribbean population and was not significant at the level of estimated rates of psychosis. Even if Black Caribbean people are more vulnerable to psychotic illnesses, the discrepancy between the data from psychiatric services and the general population suggests that they are also treated differently in the UK. Possible explanations suggested by the EMPIRIC study are racism by psychiatrists and in the community, misunderstanding of cultural expressions of distress, differential responses by police and social and treatment services and social inequality. However, why such factors should operate for Black Caribbean people and not for other ethnic minorities is not clear. The EMPIRIC results are important in illustrating how ethnic group influences a person's pathway through the health services.

Fourth, there have been two large-scale population surveys of adults and children, representative of minority ethnic groups across England – the Health Survey for England in 1999 (Erens et al, 2001) and in 2004 (Sproston and Mindell, 2006). Both surveys reveal a complex distribution of health among the major ethnic groups. While some minority ethnic groups have significantly higher rates of disease (for example, cardiovascular disease among Pakistani and Bangladeshi groups, tuberculosis and sexually transmitted infections among Black African groups), other minority ethnic groups like the Chinese have better health than the majority White population. The two surveys are especially useful for looking at trends in patterns of health by ethnic group since the Acheson Report. Although a gap of five years is a relatively short time for analysing changes in population health, the rare availability of such population-representative data on ethnic minorities in 1999 and in 2004 makes it useful to see if there has been any narrowing of the health gap between ethnic groups living in England.

As may be expected, the trends by ethnicity are complex. For some health conditions, there is little change. Among the general population and all minority ethnic groups, there was no change in the prevalence of bad or very bad self-reported general health between 1999 and 2004. The pattern for age-standardised prevalence of doctor-diagnosed diabetes among minority ethnic groups relative to the general population was the same in 2004 as in 1999, among both men and women. Overall, the patterns for obesity by ethnic group in 2004 were similar to those in 1999, although for most groups the absolute levels of overweight and obesity have increased.

For other health indicators, there is some narrowing of the health gap (for example, smoking among Irish and Black Caribbean men, and physical activity among Bangladeshi and Chinese men). However, there is also a worrying increase in poor health for some minority ethnic groups. The levels of long-standing illness and limiting long-standing illness were significantly higher for Pakistani women in 2004 than they were in 1999. There was a general increase in the prevalence of cardiovascular disease (CVD) in all minority ethnic groups between

1999 and 2004. This increase was non-significant except for Pakistani men where the prevalence of CVD doubled significantly between the two surveys (see Figure 6.1). The prevalence of hypertension was higher in 2004 than in 1999 in most minority ethnic groups, although many of the increases were not statistically significant. There was a notable reduction in regular physical activity participation among Pakistani men between 1999 and 2004. Mean C-reactive protein generally did not change for different minority ethnic groups between 1999 and 2004 except for Pakistani men, in whom a significant increase was found in the proportion of informants with high levels. Between 1999 and 2004, mean ferritin increased significantly in Pakistani and Irish men, and in Black Caribbean and Bangladeshi women. Black Caribbean women showed significant increases in both mean LDL cholesterol, and in the prevalence of raised LDL cholesterol, which is an important risk factor for cardiovascular disease.

From this heterogeneous pattern of changes in ethnic minority health from 1999 to 2004, perhaps the most consistent pattern is the widening gap between the health of the majority population and that of Pakistani men and women. This widening gap is compounded by the fact that they experience some of the poorest health in the population, and suggests that efforts to reduce the health gap between ethnic groups are not being successful, at least at the population health level.

In addition to these population representative surveys, there has been a large-scale epidemiological study of Gypsies and Travellers

**Figure 6.1: Prevalence of any cardiovascular disease by ethnic group in 1999 and 2004 among men aged 16 and over**

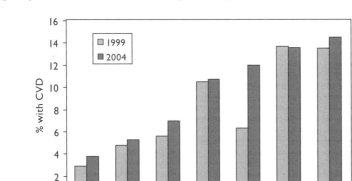

*Source:* Health Survey for England 2004 (Sproston and Mindell, 2006)

(Parry et al, 2004). Results of this quantitative survey show that Gypsy Travellers have significantly poorer health status and significantly more self-reported symptoms of ill health than other UK-resident, English-speaking ethnic minorities. Furthermore, their social circumstances are more disadvantaged compared with other ethnic groups: Gypsy and Traveller children are among the ethnic groups most eligible to receive free school meals.

The patterns of poverty, employment status and geographical location and the specifics of age structure and gender are significant in understanding the differential effects of socioeconomic position on measurable health outcomes (Cooper, 2002). Part of this differential is that some minority ethnic groups are doing better in terms of wealth and health than the ethnic majority, while others are doing considerably worse and within ethnic groups such as 'South Asian' or 'Black African' there can be considerable divergence between sub-groups. Therefore, health inequalities within ethnic groups as well as between the ethnic majority and minority groups need to be considered.

## Evidence on health service use and access

The routine recording of ethnic group was first introduced into the NHS in 1995/96. On admission to hospital, patients were asked to assign themselves to one of a list of ethnic groups matching those used in the 1991 census. The percentage of hospital inpatients with missing ethnicity was 52% in 1996/97 and 40% in 2000/01 (LHO, 2003). In 2001, the new census coding for ethnic groups was adopted and NHS hospitals were required to collect information on ethnicity in the revised format. By 2002, the proportion of hospital records with missing ethnicity coding dropped to 32%. In other NHS services, including Primary Care, Community and Mental Health Trusts, the range of ethnicity data varies hugely from 100% to just 17% (LHO, 2003). This provides a graphic illustration that some trusts can achieve high levels of valid recording, while others do not routinely collect ethnic origin data. For example, ethnic origin is not included in cancer registration data, despite higher than average incidence rates of specific cancers for men born in Scotland and Ireland (Harding and Rosato, 1999). The variable quality of these data makes monitoring of the effects of health services on mortality and morbidity inequalities very difficult. The complexity of what is meant by 'access to' and 'use of' health services has been illustrated by a case study of diabetes services in which minority ethnic patients who had access to the service could not necessarily make full use of it, nor could they assume that their healthcare needs were being met appropriately (Rhodes et al, 2003). In a prospective study of coronary disease, among patients who were suitable, South Asian patients were less likely than White patients to receive coronary artery bypass grafting (Feder et al, 2002). The differences could not be attributed to physician bias and, in the absence of any comparison of clinical outcomes, could not straightforwardly be interpreted as the result of discrimination.

Ethnicity is not at present recorded on either birth or death certificates in the United Kingdom. A proposal has been made to include ethnicity at birth and death registration in England and Wales (Aspinall et al, 2003).

## Explanations for inequalities

As well as documenting patterns of difference, there has been significant progress in establishing explanations of the patterns of health inequalities by ethnic group (see also Chapters Four and Five of this volume for a discussion of explanations of health inequality). A life-course approach has shown how the accumulation of socioeconomic disadvantage over time is related to higher risks of mortality among South Asian groups (Harding and Balarajan, 2001). The independence of the relationship between health and the experience of racism has been convincingly demonstrated (Karlsen and Nazroo, 2002). This is conceptually significant, since racism has often been assumed to be an aspect of deprivation, without a separate ill effect on health. Serious attempts to reduce behavioural risk factors for heart attack and stroke have shown the need to adopt differential strategies that emphasise different risk factors among different ethnic groups, especially in relation to alcohol use in the White population and weight in the Black Caribbean population (Dundas et al, 2001).

## Racism

The publication in 1999 of Macpherson's report on the Stephen Lawrence Inquiry brought the term 'institutional racism' to public attention, defining it as follows:

> ... the collective failure of an organisation to provide appropriate and professional service to people because of their colour, culture or ethnic origin. It can be seen or detected in processes, attitudes and behaviours which

amount to discrimination through unwitting prejudice, ignorance, thoughtlessness and racist stereotyping which disadvantage minority people. (Macpherson, 1999, para 6.34)

By highlighting institutional racism as a problem in the police force, the report also made it a matter of concern for public services in general. Despite its widespread use in terms of tackling health inequalities caused or exacerbated by institutionalised racism, Macpherson's definition is problematic because of it imprecision. This imprecision has its strategic uses, for instance in arguing that service provision failures such as inadequate translation and interpretation in the NHS can be seen as institutional racism and should be addressed and rectified (Green et al, 2002). The problem is that the documentation of how institutionalised racism operates organisationally, necessary in order to unravel its effects, is largely missing from the research literature. Instead, what can be found is the assertion of its presence due to the documentation of inequity, as in the following excerpt from a report on mental health services for minority ethnic groups that defines institutional racism as:

... a feature of institutions where there are pervasive racist attitudes and practices, assumptions based on racial differences, practices and procedures which are discriminatory in outcome, if not intent, and a tolerance or acceptance of such differences. (DH, 2003, p 37)

## 2000 Race Relations (Amendment) Act

To promote race equality in a modern, diverse Britain, the 2000 Race Relations (Amendment) Act places a general duty on public sector services, including the English, Welsh and Scottish NHS, to eliminate unlawful racial discrimination and to promote equality of opportunity and good relations between persons of different racial groups. This duty covers all aspects of an organisation's activities, policy, planning and service delivery, as well as employment practice (LHO, 2003). Furthermore, public sector organisations are required to monitor their activities for any adverse impact on race equality and demonstrate that they are making progress in race equality over a three-year period.

Requirements for ethnicity monitoring are set out in a range of NHS strategies, and yet there is little evidence of a consistent approach (LHO, 2003). A report into the implementation of the Race Relations (Amendment) Act among English strategic health authorities found wide variation in the approach taken towards race equality performance management (Bhatt, 2003). It pointed in particular to a lack of knowledge and understanding of the Act and its implications, lack of clarity about the relationship between the implementation of the Act and delivering on the modernisation agenda and *The NHS Plan* (DH, 2000), and differences in understanding of the role of health authorities in performance management of this area. Strategic health authorities tend to focus on targets related to waiting lists and times, financial balance and hospital ratings, with less priority being assigned to race equality. It cannot be assumed that NHS organisations will independently pick up on race equality areas in the future without centrally driven and sustained agenda and priority setting.

## General and specific policies

The two types of recommendations considered by the Acheson Inquiry to reduce ethnic inequalities in health – general initiatives to tackle poverty and those specifically targeted at minority ethnic people – have their own strengths and weaknesses. The task of assessing whether such policies are contributing towards the narrowing of inequalities between ethnic groups is hampered by the relative lack of robust, nationally representative data sets with appropriate measurement of ethnicity and authoritative analysis. It is only in the past few years that it has become possible to investigate ethnic inequalities in health and their structuring through social and economic disadvantage (Nazroo, 2003). Our assessment of the pattern of inequalities by ethnicity makes reference to population-representative data that have been published since the Acheson Inquiry. The inquiry confined itself to its tightly defined brief in terms of evidence surveyed and scope of recommendations. This left a number of features of ethnic minorities in Britain that were not addressed, such as religion and language, yet they may be relevant to health inequalities.

Anti-poverty and regeneration policies of the past decade have often been locality-based (for example, Sure Start, New Deal and Health Action Zones). While community ownership of state-funded policies has merit as a means of promoting engagement, the extent to which the population of impoverished people can be reached with locality-based initiatives is a problem in terms of promoting equity (see Chapter Eleven for further discussion of community-based initiatives). The difficulties of reaching people of minority ethnicity in poverty differ from those of reaching the general population because of geographic and demographic factors. The overwhelming concentration of minority groups in London and other big cities is such that rural poverty is not currently a significant issue for this group. Despite the concentration of minority ethnic groups in cities, there is little evidence of the development of neighbourhood ghettoes (Dorling and Thomas, 2004). Data from the 2001 census show that even in localities with the highest concentration they are nonetheless a minority: in Tower Hamlets 33% of the population is of Bangladeshi origin; in Leicester 26% is of Indian origin. The highest proportion of all minorities in England and Wales can be found in London, with the exception of those of Pakistani origin, who are concentrated in greatest numbers in the West Midlands and Yorkshire and Humber. So the issue of the reach of locality-based policies is problematic for minority ethnic groups, as for the ethnic majority. Anti-poverty policies are greatly needed among those minorities who suffer disproportionate levels of unemployment and material deprivation compared with others: within socioeconomic class grouping there is a minority ethnic disadvantage, particularly for people of Bangladeshi and Pakistani origin (Nazroo, 1998). The youthful age structure of minorities, especially those who migrated more recently, can exacerbate poverty because of the greater number of dependants per household.

A study by the Centre for Analysis of Social Exclusion at the London School of Economics (Hills and Stewart, 2005) has surveyed the evidence on the impact of government policies aimed at alleviating poverty, inequality and social exclusion since the Labour government was elected in 1997. The study suggests that policy responses have been variable, with certain areas such as employment, education, child poverty and neighbourhood regeneration being equipped with substantial new resources, and other areas, including the tackling of inequalities between ethnic groups, having received considerably less attention and resources. The study concluded that ethnicity was generally a sub-focus within social disadvantage, rather than the focus of specific policies. While there was a narrowing of the gap between ethnic groups in GCSE attainment (General Certificate of Secondary Education taken during the fifth year in secondary school), other dimensions of socioeconomic disadvantage such as lack of labour market participation continued to show a strong association with ethnic minority groups.

Policies specifically targeted at minority groups might offer some hope of addressing carefully defined and specific local problems with greater success than general policies; the devolution of commissioning to Primary Care Trust level makes this a current possibility. However, targeted policies are by no means a panacea and can reinforce ill-founded assumptions of homogeneity and immutability about the targeted group, which may in turn further disadvantage people who have atypical health needs. The definition of a health priority for a particular ethnic group may be used, albeit inadvertently, as a summary of that group's needs, which may subsequently feed into a stereotyped way of treating that group. An example is the Asian Mother and Baby Campaign funded by the Department of Health, which sought to address some of the adverse outcomes observed in mothers of South Asian origin and their babies by employing interpreters and link workers to undertake health advocacy roles (Parsons and Day, 1992). However, difficulties in accessing care have also been attributed to poverty and a lack of transportation (Hayes, 1995), issues that cannot be easily addressed by good interpretation services or health advocacy.

An unavoidable (and recognised) problem with the Acheson Inquiry's recommendations on ethnicity and health inequalities was the incomplete evidence base on which they drew. What is meant by ethnicity and the proxies used for its measurement has varied greatly over the past 30 years as ethnicity and health has grown as a field of research. While a question on ethnic group was asked in the 1991 census, it was amended in the 2001 census (Aspinall, 2000), when a question on religion was asked for the first time in England and Wales. The recent arrival of these questions means that statutory data offer snapshots whose validity and reliability is hard to interpret. Categories for ethnic monitoring in the NHS were modified in 2001 and the ongoing poor quality of the data does not provide a good basis for understanding inequalities in employment, service use or outcome by ethnic group. If the value of the Acheson Report is to be judged by the quality of its evidence base, the work on minority ethnic health inequalities was, inevitably, limited.

## Conclusion

The inequity of material deprivation, with well-documented ill effects on morbidity and mortality rates, can be compounded by forms of exclusion that are peculiar to minority ethnic groups. Discrimination based on religion, skin colour or an aspect of appearance such as dress that is perceived as racism may be further compounded by the deleterious effects of institutional organisations that create barriers for those who, for instance, do not speak English or who follow a special diet. Poverty, racism and various forms of discrimination operate so as to compound one another's effects and therefore it would seem that policies need to tackle the particularities of minority ethnic inequalities. However, the danger of having interventions targeted at specific minorities is that the policy is proscriptive about the culture in question and this reinforces the idea that minority cultures are bounded and static (Bradby, 2003). There is also a danger that new minorities, arriving as illegal immigrants, refugees and asylum seekers, whose culture has not yet been recognised by public services, may be excluded. Health policy should seek to embed the protection of minority ethnic health into mainstream healthcare delivery, but how this can be done with the current patchy research database and the absence of good monitoring data remains unclear. The widening health gap for some minority ethnic groups, most notably for Pakistani men, suggests that the recommendations from the Acheson Report on reducing inequalities in health between ethnic groups are not currently effective at the population health level.

## Practical steps to tackle inequalities

Since poverty and racism compound one another's effect so as to disadvantage people experiencing exclusion for reasons of material deprivation and for reasons of discrimination on grounds of poverty and racialised assumptions about difference, both have to be tackled. Ethnicity, like class and gender, is a complex, dynamic and contingent characteristic whose properties can pertain to individuals, families and larger groups. The context-dependent, labile nature of ethnicity means that a single policy to ameliorate all deficits associated with ethnicity is unlikely. However, there are two problems that affect minority ethnic groups disproportionately and never trouble the British ethnic majority in the British welfare state: first, the lack of a common language for communication with professionals; second, discrimination based on racialised ideas of difference. The lack of shared language disadvantages individuals seeking services and the availability and quality of interpretation services in the NHS is patchy, at best (Bradby, 2001). A widespread assumption that minorities should assimilate to a British norm may explain why the expense of interpretation services is often a low priority for trusts. A commitment to removing language as a barrier to accessing health services would have a significant impact on the quality of care, advice and information for people without fluent English. A translation service that was able to ensure the uptake of services and benefits by marginalised groups could have a long-term effect on the well-being of minority groups. It might also have a symbolic effect in signalling a willingness to cater for minorities on their own terms.

Racism is a separate issue, but tackling it at an institutional level would be likely to have a beneficial effect on health at the individual level. The 2000 Race Relations (Amendment) Act could aid in reducing institutional racism and its effects on the health of minority ethnic groups, but the issues are likely to vary across the UK. Nine per cent of England's population was of minority ethnicity according to the 2001 Census (including so-called mixed categories) and these people are concentrated in London. The experience of racism in London may differ considerably from Wales (where 96% of those responding to the 2001 census gave their ethnic origin as White British), Scotland (88% White Scottish) or Northern Ireland (99% gave their ethnic group as White). Whether a single piece of legislation will be effective in these different settings remains to be seen. Interpersonal racism is much harder to tackle and to legislate against. Perhaps the most practical step in tackling ethnic inequalities arising from both poverty and racism is to make sure that data on ethnicity are reliably collected and coded in all surveys.

## References

Acheson, D. (1998) *Independent inquiry into inequalities in health*, London: The Stationery Office.

Aspinall, P. (2000) 'The new 2001 census question set on cultural characteristics: is it useful for the monitoring of the health status of people from ethnic groups in Britain?', *Ethnicity and Health*, vol 5, no 1, pp 33-40.

Aspinall P.J., Jacobson, B. and Polato, G.M. (2003) *Missing record: The case for recording ethnicity at birth and death registration*, London: London Health Observatory.

Bhatt, C. (2003) 'Promoting race equality in the English NHS: a progress review', Report to the Commission for Racial Equality (http://193.113.211.175/downloads/docs/sha_report.doc).

Bhopal R. (1997) 'Is research into ethnicity and health racist, unsound, or important science?', *BMJ*, vol 314, pp 1751-6.

Bradby, H. (2001) 'Communication, interpretation and translation', in S. Dyson and L. Culley (eds) *Sociology, ethnicity and nursing*, Basingstoke: Macmillan, pp 129-48.

Bradby, H. (2003) 'Describing ethnicity in health research', *Ethnicity and Health*, vol 8, no 1, pp 5-13.

Cooper, H. (2002) 'Investigating socio-economic explanations for gender and ethnic inequalities in health', *Social Science and Medicine*, vol 54, no 4, pp 693-706.

DH (Department of Health) (2000) *The NHS Plan: A plan for investment, a plan for reform*, Cm 4818, London: The Stationery Office.

DH (2003) *Inside outside: Improving mental health services for black and minority ethnic communities in England*, London: The Stationery Office.

Dorling, D. and Thomas, B. (2004) *People and places: A 2001 Census atlas of the UK*, Bristol: The Policy Press.

Dundas, R., Morgan, M., Redfern, J., Lemic-Stojcevic, N. and Wolfe, C. (2001) 'Ethnic differences in behavioural risk factors for stroke: implications for health promotion', *Ethnicity and Health*, vol 6, no 2, pp 95-104.

Erens, B., Primatesta, P. and Prior, G. (eds) (2001) *Health Survey for England 1999: The health of minority ethnic groups. Vol 1: Findings. Vol 2: Methodology and documentation*, London: The Stationery Office.

Feder, G., Crook, A.M., Magee, P., Banerjee, S., Timmis, A.D. and Hemingway, H. (2002) 'Ethnic differences in invasive management of coronary disease: prospective cohort study of patients undergoing angiography', *BMJ*, vol 324, pp 511-16.

Green, G., Bradby, H., Chan, A., Lee, M. and Eldridge, K. (2002) 'Equity and culture: is the NHS failing to meet the needs of mentally distressed Chinese origin women in England?', *Journal of Health Services Research and Policy*, vol 7, no 4, pp 216-21.

Harding, S. and Balarajan, R. (2000) 'Limiting long-term illness among Black Caribbeans, Black Africans, Indians, Pakistanis, Bangladeshis and Chinese born in the UK', *Ethnicity and Health*, vol 5, no 1, pp 41-6.

Harding, S. and Balarajan, R. (2001) 'Longitudinal study of socio-economic differences in mortality among South Asian and West Indian migrants', *Ethnicity and Health*, vol 6, no 2, pp 121-8.

Harding, S. and Rosato, M. (1999) 'Cancer incidence among first generation Scottish, Irish, West Indian and South Asian migrants living in England and Wales', *Ethnicity and Health*, vol 4, no 1/2, pp 83-92.

Harding, S., Rosato, M.J. and Cruikshank, J.K. (2004) 'Lack of change in birthweights of infants by generational status among Indian, Pakistani, Bangladeshi, Black Caribbean, and Black African mothers in a British cohort study', *International Journal of Epidemiology*, vol 33, no 6, pp 1279-85.

Hayes, L. (1995) 'Unequal access to midwifery care: a continuing problem', *Journal of Advanced Nursing*, vol 21, no 4, pp 702-7.

Hills, J. and Stewart, K. (eds) (2005) *A more equal society? New Labour, poverty, inequality and exclusion*, Bristol: The Policy Press.

Karlsen, S. and Nazroo, J. (2002) 'Relation between racial discrimination, social class, and health among ethnic minority groups', *American Journal of Public Health*, vol 92, no 4, pp 624-31.

LHO (London Health Observatory) (2003) *Ethnic health intelligence in London: The story so far*, London: LHO (www.lho.org.uk/HEALTH_ INEQUALITIES/EHIP/EthnicHealthIntelligence.aspx).

Macpherson, W. (1999) *The Stephen Lawrence Inquiry: Report of an inquiry by Sir William Macpherson of Cluny*, Cm 4262-I, London: The Stationery Office (www.archive.official-documents.co.uk/document/ cm42/4262/sli-06.htm).

Nazroo, J.Y. (1998) 'Genetic, cultural or socio-economic vulnerability? Explaining ethnic inequalities in health', *Sociology of Health and Illness*, vol 20, no 5, pp 710-30.

Nazroo, J.Y. (2003) 'The structuring of ethnic inequalities in health: economic position, racial discrimination and racism', *American Journal of Public Health*, vol 93, no 2, pp 277-85.

ONS (Office for National Statistics) (2005) *Focus on ethnicity*, London: ONS (www.statistics.gov.uk/downloads/theme_compendia/ foe2004/Ethnicity.pdf).

Parry, G., Van Cleemput, P., Peters, J., Moore, J., Walters, S., Thomas, K. and Cooper, C. (2004) *Health status of Gypsies and Travellers in England*, Report of Department of Health Inequalities in Health Research initiative, Sheffield: School of Health and Related Research, University of Sheffield.

Parsons, L. and Day, S. (1992) 'Improving obstetric outcomes in ethnic minorities: an evaluation of health advocacy in Hackney', *Journal of Public Health Medicine*, vol 14, no 2, pp 183-91.

Rhodes, P., Nocon, A., and Wright, J. (2003) 'Access to diabetes services: the experiences of Bangladeshi people in Bradford, UK', *Ethnicity and Health*, vol 8, no 3, pp 171-88.

Sproston, K. and Nazroo, J. (2002) *Ethnic minority psychiatric illness rates in the community (EMPIRIC): Quantitative report*, London: The Stationery Office (www.doh.gov.uk/public/empiric.htm).

Sproston, K. and Mindell, J. (2006) *Health Survey for England 2004. Vol 1: The health of minority ethnic groups*, London: National Centre for Social Research.

# SEVEN

# Housing conditions and health

*David Ormandy*

## Introduction

There are some very obvious wide differences in housing. This chapter largely deals with conditions in the UK, particularly in England, because of the availability of data and the policy changes that have occurred. However, the principles and discussions can be applied elsewhere in the UK. There are differences in housing archetypes – detached, semi-detached, terraced, maisonettes and flats, and houses in multiple occupation; and differences in housing age, which for the purposes of this chapter reflect major changes to the building control requirements – pre-1920, 1920-45, 1946-79, post-1979. There are differences of location – urban, rural, north of England, south of England; differences in tenure – freehold, leasehold, commonhold, private sector tenancies, public sector tenancies, and licences; and differences in access to housing – financial resources and qualifying status (need and vulnerability).

Some of these differences may reflect or influence inequalities: the most obvious are the value of the dwelling as an asset, the security of tenure and the socioeconomic status of the occupants. Some differences may have a direct or indirect impact on health: housing type and age, tenure and condition. This chapter concentrates on the potential effect of housing conditions on health, and on how other factors influence the impact on health that may lead to inequalities, including policies and actions following the recommendations made by the Acheson Inquiry (Acheson, 1998). These recommendations included improving the quality of housing and, specifically, actions to address fuel poverty, accidental (unintentional) home injuries, fire safety and fear of crime.

It is now accepted that housing conditions affect health, and, particularly, that unsatisfactory conditions can have a negative impact on health. However, while the evidence base is considerable and growing, and a strong association between housing and health outcomes has been well established, there are major methodological challenges in trying to unravel the potential impact of individual and combinations of housing conditions from other environmental, social and economic factors. What is also clear is that the more vulnerable members of society are more likely to be exposed to the worst and most health-threatening conditions.

The chapter begins with a discussion of definitions of housing and of health, and follows with evidence on the relationship between housing conditions and health, especially that which supports the contention that it is the most vulnerable sectors of society that are most at risk. Where appropriate, the policies and practices that have influenced housing, primarily housing conditions and tenure, and, in particular, the changes over the past 10 years, will be discussed.

## Housing and health: definitions

Housing is fundamental to everyday life and represents more than just the physical structure, but what that representation means is not always clear. Here the term 'house' is used to indicate a particular type of dwelling, and a 'dwelling' is used to mean the physical structure (or part of a structure) that is used, or intended to be used, for human habitation. Too often the terms 'house' and 'home' are used as synonyms, but the word 'home' more correctly describes the social, cultural and economic structure established by the occupants. 'Housing' includes more than just the single dwelling and its occupants; it includes the neighbourhood and the community, the 'neighbourhood' being the streets or estate and their infrastructure in which the dwelling is situated and the 'community' including the other residents, and those servicing the neighbourhood. So, the dwelling and the neighbourhood could be thought of as the 'hardware', and the home and the community the 'software', with the term 'housing' being used to embrace all four elements.

Housing should provide a safe and healthy environment, should allow for family life, for privacy, and for social interaction with friends, relatives and members of the community. As such, the most appropriate definition of health in relation to housing is that proposed by the World Health Organization – 'a state of complete physical, mental and social well-being and not merely the absence of disease or infirmity' (WHO, 1952). But we want and need things that are potential hazards in our dwellings: stairs and steps, windows, doors, means of heating for the space and for water, cooking facilities, gas and electricity. So, while our dwellings cannot be guaranteed completely safe, any necessary and unavoidable hazards should be as safe as possible, and dwellings should be designed and constructed to take account of the spectrum of lifestyles that may typically occupy them.

# Dwelling conditions in relation to health
## The evidence base

Over the past 20 years, there has been an increasing interest in gathering and strengthening evidence on the relationship between housing and health. This has included revising and updating evidence on building conditions and the health of users (Mant and Muir Gray, 1986; Cox and O'Sullivan, 1995; Raw and Hamilton, 1995; Raw et al, 2001) and several reviews on housing and health (for example, Ranson, 1991; Ineichan, 1993; Burridge and Ormandy, 1993; AJPH, 2003; BMA, 2003; Howden-Chapman and Carroll, 2004; RenvH, 2004). There have also been several conferences that have demonstrated the wealth of international studies, including a series of Unhealthy Housing conferences at the University of Warwick, in 1986, 1987, 1991 and 2003 and the World Health Organization's symposiums on Housing and Health in 2002 and 2004.

## Potential hazards from dwelling conditions

Work commissioned by the UK government in 2003 offered a further opportunity to build on the previous reviews of research linking dwelling conditions with health and safety (ODPM, 2003a). This work also included the analysis of matched databases – a Housing and Population Database and datasets on reported illness, injuries and other health conditions – to provide information on the prevalence of a wide range of illness, injuries and other health conditions linked to housing conditions in England. The analyses identified 29 potential hazards, shown in Table 7.1, all of which were attributable, to a greater or lesser extent, to dwelling design and/or condition.

In other words, no one hazard, such as environmental tobacco smoke, was attributable solely to occupier behaviour. Initial estimates suggested that, in England, these hazards were implicated in up to 50,000 deaths and around 0.5 million injuries and illnesses requiring medical attention each year. It was also found that accidents in the home (whether through carelessness or otherwise) resulted in more injuries than accidents at work or on the road, as shown in Table 7.2.

Further analyses were carried out to identify, for each of the 29 hazards, whether any particular age group of the population was more vulnerable than others, and also whether a hazard was more likely to occur in any particular age band of property.

**Table 7.1: Potential housing hazards**

| Physiological requirements | Protection against infection |
|---|---|
| Damp and mould growth, etc | Domestic hygiene, pests and refuse |
| Excessive cold | Food safety |
| Excessive heat | Personal hygiene, sanitation and |
| Asbestos, etc |   drainage |
| Biocides | Water supply |
| CO and fuel combustion |   |
|   productions | **Protection against accidents** |
| Lead | Falls associated with baths, etc |
| Radiation | Falling on level surfaces |
| Uncombusted fuel gas | Falling on stairs, etc |
| Volatile organic compounds | Falling between levels |
|   | Electrical hazards |
| **Psychological requirements** | Fire |
| Crowding and space | Flames, hot surfaces, etc |
| Entry by intruders | Collision and entrapment |
| Lighting | Explosions |
| Noise | Position and operability of |
|   |   amenities, etc |
|   | Structural collapse and falling |
|   |   elements |

Based on ODPM (2006a)

**Table 7.2: Deaths and injuries from accidents at home, at work and on the road (England and Wales)**

|  | Accidental | | Total accidents |
|---|---|---|---|
|  | Deaths | Injuries |  |
| Road (2002) | 3,431 | 299,174 | 302,605 |
| Work (12 months during 2002/03) | 235* | 154,430 | 154,665 |
| Home and garden (2002) | 3,000** | 2,701,326 | 2,704,326 |

\* 2003/04 figures.
\*\* Official estimate.
Based on data from Royal Society for Prevention of Accidents, Health and Safety Executive, and Department of Trade and Industry Home Accident Surveillance System

## The cost of unhealthy dwellings

As well as the direct effect on the individual concerned, negative health outcomes from dwelling conditions have a cost to society. There is the obvious direct cost to the health service, but there are also indirect costs incurred by the victim's household, and the cost to society of any state benefits to which the victim is subsequently entitled. Recent research has tried to quantify the total economic burden of illness and other health conditions attributable to housing (Ambrose, 2001, 2005), although there are difficulties in apportioning such costs. There has also been some work on the cost of accidental injuries in the home. One recent study, in the Netherlands, estimated that home injuries cost around €0.66 billion (£0.45 billion) in healthcare costs alone (Meerding et al, 2006), and another recent study, in the US, estimated that the total cost to society[1] of accidental home injuries was at least $217 billion (£149 billion), made up of $1.74 million (£1.19 million) per fatal injury and $288,000 (£197,500) for each hospital-admitted non-fatal injury (Zaloshnja et al, 2005).

## Housing tenure in England

Between 1914 and 1996, the private rented sector in England shrank from 89% to a mere 9%, while the owner-occupied sector grew from 19% to 69% over the same period. The public sector share of the stock (local authority and registered social landlords) also increased, from 1% in 1914 to 22% in 1996 (DETR, 1998a). There were several factors at play over this period, including landlords selling off housing as rent controls depressed the investment returns and the growth of the public sector providing an alternative to the private sector. In addition, the 1980 Housing Act gave public sector tenants the 'right to buy' their dwelling at a discount, increasing owner-occupation at the expense of the public sector. The result was that by 2001, although the number of dwellings had increased, 70% of the housing stock was owner-occupied, 10% rented from private landlords, 13% rented from local authorities and 7% rented from registered social landlords (ODPM, 2003b).

## Dwelling standards

For at least 150 years, there has been some form of acknowledgement of the relationship between health and dwelling conditions underlying the English housing standards, although by the 1990s this had become obscured. In the early 19th century, there was considerable pressure for a recognition that the 'market' would do nothing to maintain or drive up housing standards because of the imbalance in the relationship between landlord and tenant. This led to a demand for some form of state intervention to ensure that, at the very least, the perceived causes of disease were eliminated. This movement promoted what became known as the 'sanitary idea', built on a notion that smells were linked with disease, and that diseases were spread by 'miasma' (Finer, 1952). The theory as put into practice was to remove the sources of smells – rubbish, raw sewage – and make provision for fresh air and light, and the incidence of diseases would be reduced. The diseases, and the problems, were concentrated in the crowded rookeries housing the 'labouring population'. Although we know now that this theory was built on a flawed notion, the solutions adopted were relatively effective in removing some of the more blatant threats to health.

There were, and still are, two regulatory approaches adopted to deal with insanitary or unhealthy housing. One was to create standards and requirements to control the design and construction of *new* dwellings; the other was to impose standards on all *existing* dwellings (those occupied or available for occupation). Originally, controls on new dwellings were through byelaws adopted by local authorities, but since the 1960s, these have been replaced by national building regulations. While these regulations have been updated regularly to try to ensure that modern dwellings provide a relatively safe and healthy residential environment, new dwellings are in fact a very small minority of the housing stock – in 2001, of the 21.1 million dwellings in England, only about 6% were relatively new (ODPM, 2003b). In fact, over a third (39%) of the English housing stock was built before 1945, and over a fifth (21%) before 1919. As renewal of the existing stock is a very gradual process (and at the current rate of replacement, it will take more than 160 years), there is still a need for controls on existing housing to try to ensure that it is as free as possible from threats to health and safety.

The first suggestions for a national (English) minimum standard for existing housing were made in 1919 (Ministry of Health, 1919), but it was not until 1954 that a national definition was introduced into the legislation in the form of the Housing Repairs and Rents Act. This definition listed eight general and basic requirements that had to be satisfied for a dwelling to be considered fit for human habitation, including the state of repair, dampness, natural lighting, water supply, sanitary conveniences and cooking facilities. With only two minor changes, this remained the national standard for the next 36 years. It was replaced by the 1989 Local Government and Housing Act, which was really just an update of the 1954 version, although it did introduce for the first time requirements for the provision of artificial lighting, for heating, hot water and personal washing facilities.

Although there may have been some public health principles underlying the English standards for housing, the phrasing has always been more focused on buildings – the condition of the structure and the presence of basic amenities. This has meant that the extent or cost of the remedial works had a strong if not overriding influence on assessments of the seriousness of housing conditions, rather than the potential impact on health.

## Action to deal with unsatisfactory dwellings

Where a dwelling was identified as failing the fitness standard, a duty was placed on local authorities to intervene, either to ensure that it was made fit or that it was no longer available for occupation (that is, it was closed). These powers can be traced back to 1936 at least, and remained largely unchanged until 2006. The duties were not tenure-specific: they applied whether the dwelling was privately or publicly owned, and whether it was owner-occupied or tenanted. However, local authorities are unable to take action against themselves, and, as far as possible, have avoided taking action against owner-occupiers.

Financial aid, in the form of grant aid and, to some extent, loans, has been available towards the cost of repairs and improvement. At various times, the criteria and conditions relating to financial aid have changed. At one time, determining that a dwelling was unfit automatically qualified the owner (whether landlord or occupier) as eligible for grant aid (although the actual amount was means-tested). At other times, priorities and qualifying criteria were at the discretion of the local authority.

## Dwelling conditions and inequalities

To state the obvious, one aim of any standard or regulation is to protect those most likely to be exposed to possible threats. In the case of dwellings, the prime intention is to protect the residents, and those who make the most use of, and place most demands on, housing include some of the most vulnerable of society. While many of us spend at least eight to 12 hours a day at home, the very young, the elderly, the unemployed and those who are ill or otherwise not healthy enough to go to work or school may spend up to 24 hours a day in and around the dwelling. Therefore any system for regulating housing conditions should be directed to protecting the main users, and if a dwelling is safe for these, the more vulnerable, it will be safe for all.

Since the late 1950s, although the legislation has not singled out any particular group, the minimum standards for housing were set so low as to focus only on the very worst conditions: that is, conditions most likely to be suffered by those with the least options, with few resources, and with the least control over their housing. Those in a position to do so choose better-quality housing. This view is supported by data from the 1996 English House Condition Survey (EHCS) (DETR, 1998a). In 1996, of the 20.4 million dwellings in England, more than 1.5 million (7.5%) were considered unfit. Most of these (1.2 million) were in the private sector: 19.3% of private rented housing and only 6% of owner-occupied dwellings were deemed unfit. Not surprisingly, it was the older houses where the worst conditions were concentrated, with nearly 50% of unfit houses being built before 1919. Households where the household head was unemployed were more likely to live in unfit housing (17%) than the employed (5%); and 20% of the 2.4 million elderly households lived in poor housing.[2] The survey also found that private sector tenants were more likely to be in poor housing (31%), and that, of those, 41% were receiving housing benefit and 47% were unemployed. As there was some underlying health basis for the fitness standard, the EHCS supports the contention that it was the more vulnerable sectors of the community that were exposed to conditions likely to threaten their health.

## Recent policies and housing

Over the past 15-20 years, there has been an insidious weakening of the security of tenure of tenants. Before then, most tenants in both the public and private sector had reasonable security: they could not be lawfully evicted without good reason. This changed in January 1989, when the Rent Act Secure and Regulated Tenancies were replaced by the Assured and Assured Shorthold Tenancies.[3] Subsequent changes, supposedly to free up the private rented sector, have meant that shorthold, usually for a six-month period, is now the most common form of tenancy. The government's housing White Paper stated that this policy was aimed at encouraging the private rented sector:

> Rent controls have prevented property owners from getting an adequate return on their investment. People who might have been prepared to grant a temporary letting have also been deterred by laws on security of tenure which make

it impossible to regain possession of their property when necessary.... Yet ... private renting offers a good option for people who need mobility ... [and] can offer greater flexibility and responsiveness to market demand. (DoE, 1987)

This 'deregulation' of the rented sector, together with the 'right to buy' policies, had dramatic effects. While there were (and still are) responsibilities placed on landlords (1961 Housing Act and 1985 Landlord and Tenant Act) to keep their properties in repair, the lack of security means that tenants are either unlikely to feel secure enough to challenge recalcitrant landlords, or are relatively transient and so unlikely to bother. The 'right to buy' at discounted prices encouraged many to buy their house, comparing their putative mortgage repayment with their rent, and not necessarily taking into account the cost of maintenance and replacement. Misjudging the cost of home ownership often resulted in 'new' low-income owner-occupiers finding they could not maintain their property or, at worst, could not meet the repayments.

The increasing imbalance between landlords and tenants meant that the only safeguard to maintaining and driving up standards in the private rented sector was reliance on the will and activities of local authorities using their powers to deal with unsatisfactory conditions. However, for the low-income owner-occupiers in unfit properties, grant aid was available towards the cost of repairs and improvements.

## A health-based housing assessment methodology

In the 1990s, and unrelated to any policy specifically directed at 'health', the (then) Department of the Environment (DoE) decided to set in train a major reform of the approach to assessing housing conditions. Various research projects were commissioned, including work on health and safety risks from housing conditions (Cox and O'Sullivan, 1995; Raw and Hamilton, 1995) and an investigation into the legal controls on existing housing in England (Ormandy et al, 1998). Ormandy and colleagues' report called for the fitness standard to be extended to cover energy efficiency, fire safety, dangerous design features and air quality, and also recommended major reform to the legal controls by developing an approach that ranked the severity of housing conditions in terms of the threats to health and safety. Based on responses to a consultation paper on proposals and options for changes to the statutory minimum standard for existing housing (DETR, 1998b), the government commissioned work to develop a health-based risk assessment approach to the appraisal of housing conditions.

This development work included reviewing the evidence, looking first at reported research on the relationship between dwelling conditions and health and safety to identify housing hazards and their potential for harm. As mentioned previously, a second stage was to match and analyse data on health outcomes with data on housing conditions (ODPM, 2003a). This second stage, producing the statistical evidence to support a housing health and safety rating system (HHSRS), highlighted whether, for each hazard, there was any particular age group more vulnerable to that hazard than the rest of the population.

Thus the concept of the HHSRS (ODPM, 2006a) was developed and tested, and it was adopted in April 2006 as the prescribed method for the assessment of housing conditions under the 2004 Housing Act, replacing the 1990 housing fitness standard.[4] The HHSRS shifts the emphasis of the assessment, and focuses on potential threats to the health and safety of users – the effects of defects. This means that conditions are judged not in terms of the cost or extent of remedial works necessary, but in terms of the severity of the threat to residents. Linked to this assessment methodology, the 2004 Act sets out an enforcement regime, providing a range of legal tools to enable local authorities to take action to protect the health and safety of residents by ensuring housing hazards are made as safe as possible.

## Decent homes

In 1997, the government introduced the decent homes standard. This is an administrative target standard. It is the government's declared aim that all public sector housing and all private sector housing occupied by 'vulnerable' individuals should meet the decent homes standard by 2010 (ODPM, 2005). For these purposes, 'vulnerability' is defined as households in receipt of pension credits or those receiving certain state benefits.[5] A 'decent home' (ODPM, 2004) is one that meets the following four requirements: that it meets the current minimum standard for housing;[6] is in a reasonable state of repair; has reasonably modern facilities; and provides a reasonable degree of thermal comfort.

In 2003, of the 21.3 million dwellings in England (ODPM, 2006b), 6.7 million failed to meet the decent homes standard: 30% of the private sector stock and 35% of the public sector stock. There was a greater percentage of 'non-decent' homes in the private rented sector (48% of the 2.2 million dwellings) than in the owner-occupied or public sectors, and of the 5.3 million private sector dwellings failing the decent homes standard, 37% were occupied by 'vulnerable' households.[7]

The 2003 EHCS (ODPM, 2006b) also reports that households with low income are more likely to live in 'non-decent' homes. There is a similar pattern for other so-called 'at risk' household groups, including households headed by someone unemployed, lone parents, those with illness or disability, those aged 60+ and those aged 75+. As mentioned previously, financial assistance towards the cost of repairs and improvement has been available through local authorities. However, the budgets for this facility have gone up and down, and there have never been sufficient funds available to satisfy the EHCS estimate of an average of £7,560 per dwelling needed to make all non-decent owner-occupied dwellings 'decent'.

## Cold homes and fuel poverty

One of the criticisms of the housing fitness standard was that it did not effectively cover energy efficiency. While the 1990 fitness standard introduced (for the first time) a requirement for the provision of heating (1985 Housing Act), government guidance stated that this could be satisfied by 'a suitably located (13 amp minimum) outlet which may reasonably be dedicated solely to [a fixed electric heating] appliance' (DoE, 1996, Annex A, para 7.4). There was no reference to thermal insulation or energy efficiency.

Although this was a very minimal standard, not concerned with matters of quality or comfort, the 2001 EHCS (ODPM, 2003b) found that 4.2% of the English housing stock failed to meet the fitness standard, and of these, just over 10% failed on heating. That means that in 2001 there were over 88,500 dwellings in England that did not meet the appallingly low requirement of a dedicated 13-amp power socket in the living room.

Responding to pressure from various quarters, the government set up the Warm Front initiative (Defra, 2000), directed at tackling fuel poverty. This, together with the decent homes programme, should go some way towards relieving some of the inequalities associated with cold homes. However, the scale of the problem is such that these two initiatives are really only the starting point.

The energy efficiency of dwellings is covered by the HHSRS, where one of the hazards to be assessed is 'excess cold'. During work on the development of the HHSRS, Moore estimated that there may be more than six million dwellings (28% of the total stock) where this hazard was at an unacceptable level (Moore, 2003). He also estimated that of these, nearly 4.5 million dwellings (that is, over one fifth of the total stock) are occupied by 'vulnerable' households.

## The future

The initiative behind the changes in housing policy that resulted in the development and introduction of the HHSRS came from the housing policy side of government, the (now) Department for Communities and Local Government (DCLG),[8] with virtually no input from the health policy side. However, the introduction of the HHSRS has in fact gone further than the policy recommendations of the report of the Acheson Inquiry (1998). The latter included a general recommendation to improve the quality of housing and specifically to adopt policies to improve thermal efficiency, reduce accidents and reduce deaths from fires. In relation to housing conditions, the adoption of the HHSRS also meets the acknowledgement at the Fourth Ministerial Conference on Environment and Health (WHO, 2005, pp 16-17) that 'Environment and health had to be at the core of policies on housing and energy use'.

There is already clear evidence of the potential negative effect housing conditions can have on the health and safety of residents, and the evidence base is growing. There is also evidence that the more vulnerable members of society are more likely to occupy unsatisfactory housing, and so be exposed to the more dangerous conditions. But not only are they more vulnerable physically, they are also more likely to be disadvantaged and less likely to be in a position to change their circumstances to avoid or remove the potential threats.

With health at the centre of the assessment of dwelling conditions, there is an opportunity for the health services and local authorities to work together, identifying priorities and monitoring the effectiveness of interventions. For example, local or regional data could be used to identify particular health and safety issues relating to housing conditions, such as fall injuries, and local authorities could target fall-related housing hazards. One example of such an approach is Bristol City Council's use of local information on burglary (covered by the HHSRS as 'entry by intruders') to inform policies, allowing local authority officers to target more vulnerable households and dwellings (Roderick, 2005). Another is the study commissioned to assess the impact of Sheffield Homes'[9] £669 million Decent Homes Programme on the health of residents. This study used the HHSRS to estimate the reduction in risk resulting from the improvement works to the 48,000 dwellings within Sheffield Homes' remit, and also the reduction in the numbers of residents that could suffer some harm sufficient to make demands on the health services (Gilbertson et al, 2006).

The introduction of the HHSRS and the associated enforcement regime provides a new set of tools for local housing authorities to attack the problems. But if they do, it will be the owners of some of the older and more dilapidated houses who will have to provide most of the funding for the works necessary. So, while the scale of the problem is clear, and the legal tools are now available, there still needs to be a political commitment, and an economic solution.

## Notes

[1] This includes costs to victims, families, government, insurers and taxpayers.

[2] The 1996 EHCS defined the term 'poor housing' as including housing that was unfit, that required substantial repairs and was in need of essential modernisation.

[3] Part 1, 1988 Housing Act.

[4] 2005 Housing Health and Safety Rating System (England) Regulations.

[5] A household where the head and/or any partner is in receipt of any of the following benefits: income support, income-based jobseeker's allowance, housing benefit, working families tax credit, disabled person's tax credit, disability living allowance – care component, disability living allowance – mobility component, industrial injuries disablement benefit, war disablement pension or attendance allowance.

[6] Until April 2006, the fitness standard was the minimum standard for housing, but on the introduction of the housing health and safety rating system (see text), the first requirement was changed to the dwelling being free of any unacceptable hazard.

[7] See note 5.

[8] The Department for Communities and Local Government was created on 5 May 2006 with a remit to promote community cohesion and equality, as well as having responsibility for housing, urban regeneration, planning and local government (see www.communities.gov.uk).

[9] The housing association managing Sheffield's public sector housing stock.

# References

Acheson, D. (1998) *Independent inquiry into inequalities in health*, London: The Stationery Office.

AJPH (*American Journal of Public Health*) (2003) Special issue: Built environment and health, vol 93, no 9.

Ambrose, P., (2001) 'Living conditions and health promotion strategies', *Journal of the Royal Society for the Promotion of Health*, vol 121, no 1, pp 9–15.

Ambrose, P. (2005) 'The health and other costs generated by poor housing', Proceedings of conference 'Habitat Insalubre et Santé', Paris, 20–21 May.

BMA (British Medical Association) (2003) *Housing and health: building for the future*, London: BMA.

Burridge, R. and Ormandy, D. (1993) *Unhealthy housing: Research, remedies and reform*, London: E & FN Spon.

Cox, S.J. and O'Sullivan, E.F.O. (eds) (1995) *Building regulation and safety*, Watford: Building Research Establishment.

Defra (Department for Environment, Food and Rural Affairs) (2000) 'Warm front' (www.defra.gov.uk/environment/energy/hees/, accessed 1 September 2006) (see also (2004) *Fuel poverty in England: The Government's plan for action*, London: Defra).

DETR (Department of the Environment, Transport and the Regions) (1998a) *English House Condition Survey 1996*, London: DETR.

DETR (1998b) *Housing fitness standard: Consultation paper*, London: DETR.

DoE (Department of the Environment) (1987) *Housing: The government's proposal*, Cm 214, London: HMSO.

DoE (1996) *Private sector renewal: A strategic approach*, Circular 17/96, London: DoE.

Finer, S.E. (1952) *The life and times of Sir Edwin Chadwick*, London: Methuen.

Gilbertson, J., Green, G. and Ormandy, D. (2006) *Decent homes: Better health*, Sheffield: Centre for Regional Economic and Social Research.

Howden-Chapman, P. and Carroll, P. (2004) *Housing and health: Research, policy and innovation*, Wellington: Steele Roberts.

Ineichen, B. (1993) *Homes and health: How housing and health interact*, London: E & FN Spon.

Mant, D. and Muir Gray, J.A. (1986) *Building regulation and health*, Watford: Building Research Establishment.

Meerding, W.J., Mulder, S. and van Beeck, E.F. (2006) Incidence and costs of injuries in the Netherlands, *European Journal of Public Health*, vol 16, no 3, pp 217-77.

Ministry of Health (1919) *Manual of unfit houses and unhealthy areas*, London: Ministry of Health.

Moore, R. (2003), Private communication.

ODPM (Office of the Deputy Prime Minister) (2003a) *Statistical evidence to support the housing health and safety rating system: Vols I, II, and III*, London: ODPM.

ODPM (2003b) *English House Condition Survey 2001*, London: ODPM.

ODPM (2004) *A decent home: The definition and guidance for implementation*, London: ODPM.

ODPM (2005) *Public Sector Service Agreement Target 7*, London: ODPM (www.communities.gov.uk/index.asp?id=1152136, accessed 20 June 2006).

ODPM (2006a) *Housing health and safety rating system: Operating guidance*, London: ODPM.

ODPM (2006b) *English House Condition Survey 2003*, London: ODPM.

Ormandy, D., Burridge, R., Raw, G. and Cayless, S. (1998) *Controlling minimum standards in existing housing*, Coventry: Legal Research Institute.

Ranson, R. (1991) *Healthy housing: A practical guide*, London: E & FN Spon.

Raw, G.J. and Hamilton, R.M. (eds) (1995) *Building regulations and health*, Watford: Building Research Establishment.

Raw, G.J., Aizlewood, C.E. and Hamilton, R.M. (eds) (2001) *Building regulation, health and safety*, Watford: Building Research Establishment.

RenvH (*Reviews on Environmental Health*) (2004) Special issue: Housing, health and well-being, vol 19, no 3-4.

Roderick, M. (2005) *Housing health and safety rating system: Hazard 12 – Entry by intruders: A local evaluation of the hazard*, Bristol: Bristol City Council.

WHO (World Health Organization) (1952) *Preamble to constitution*, Geneva: WHO.

WHO (2005) *Fourth Ministerial Conference on Environment and Health. Final report*, Copenhagen: WHO Regional Office for Europe.

Zaloshnja, E., Miller, T.R., Lawrence, B.A. and Romano, E. (2005) 'The cost of unintentional home injuries', *American Journal of Preventive Medicine*, vol 28, no 1, pp 88-94.

# EIGHT

# Inequalities in food and nutrition: challenging 'lifestyles'

*Elizabeth Dowler, Martin Caraher and Paul Lincoln*

This chapter examines work on inequalities in food and nutrition in the UK since the late 1990s, looking at how problems have been constructed and measured, responses by government and civil society, and future challenges. It begins by summarising data on social inequalities in food and nutritional intakes and outcomes, focusing largely on income and occupationally based inequalities, and outlines why these outcomes are thought to occur. The relationship with health, and particularly health inequalities, is briefly discussed. The location of the Acheson Inquiry within the food and nutrition policy context of the time, and developments since, are discussed in terms of their potential effectiveness and relevance to reducing inequalities. The chapter concludes with an outline of contemporary anxieties and activities in relation to inequalities in food and nutrition.

## Inequalities in food and nutrition

It has long been recognised that food patterns, nutrient intakes and physical outcomes of growth and attained body size vary by indicators of social and economic conditions. People who are better off are more likely to eat more healthily than those who are poorer, although the size of differences between classes varies by country (Roos et al, 1999; Dowler, 2001; Drewnowski and Specter, 2004) and may be attenuating over time (Crotty and Germov, 2004).

In the UK, differentials in household or individual dietary patterns, nutrient intake and blood levels by various socioeconomic indicators have been observed in the annual national surveys of household intakes (published by the Ministry for Agriculture, Fisheries and Food until 2000, now by Defra, the Department for Environment, Food and Rural Affairs), and in regular national surveys of individual intakes (Gregory et al, 1995; Finch, 1998; Gregory, 2000; Hoare et al, 2004). Intakes of vitamins, minerals and dietary fibre, and consumption of vegetables and (especially) fruit, are much lower (and for nutrients, further below

Reference Nutrient Intakes) and consumption of white bread, processed meats and sugar are higher in households whose members are poorer than in those whose members are more affluent (Dowler et al, 2001a). (The further a group's nutrient intake is from the reference level, the more likely it is that some members of the group have inadequate intakes that contribute to poor functioning and ill health.) The differentials are true for all age groups and geographical regions, and, in contrast with other rich industrialised countries, worsened during the 1980s and 1990s. They are particularly marked when intakes and food patterns are compared by household income, economic activity (employed versus unemployed/receiving state benefits) or household composition (Defra, 2006; Wrieden et al, 2006). Lone-parent households and those with two or more adults and children, which in the UK are more likely to be poor, are also more likely to have lower micro-nutrient intakes (Defra, 2006). In other words, nutritional inequalities in the UK were more often found to be associated with poverty and deprivation than with social class defined by occupational group or educational status. There are also differentials by minority ethnic group status, but in the main these are more likely to be associated with material and social conditions than with cultural practice.

One problem with using national survey data to look at inequalities is the small sample size for households in poor material circumstances; this is being addressed through a national survey of nutrition and diet in low-income households to be published in 2007 by the Food Standards Agency. Considerable detail about household income and other social circumstances will be available, as well as nutritional data from members of the same household. This survey will provide data to be used alongside standard representative national surveillance data to investigate more fully the nature of nutritional inequalities. Such quantitative data can be complemented by qualitative data rich in insight on cultural practice, beliefs and behavioural dynamics (for example, Dobson et al, 1994; Christie et al, 2002). Smaller-scale quantitative and qualitative surveys have hitherto been the primary source of understanding how people manage on low incomes in terms of practice and consequence. For instance, a survey of lone-parent households' diets, carried out in the early 1990s when such households' incomes were particularly likely to be low, showed that those in receipt of state benefits for more than a year, especially those repaying rent or fuel arrears (not uncommon), had half the nutrient intakes of parents not living in such circumstances. Parents' intakes of key micro-nutrients were well below reference levels, although their children's intakes were less affected (Dowler et al, 2001a). Their dietary patterns were characteristically monotonous and with little commodity variety: people mostly ate from a small range of foods or composite dishes. Such findings highlight the realities of living on low income for long periods and the effect on food expenditure, and were independent of other sociodemographic indicators, including smoking and self-defined ethnic group.

As well as food patterns and nutrient intakes, nutritional outcome indicators of body size are strongly socially patterned: women, and, increasingly, men and children, from lower socioeconomic groups are more likely to be obese or overweight, or (in children) thin and short for their age (Gregory, 2000; Wardle et al, 2002; Drewnowski and Specter, 2004; HC, 2004; Hoare et al, 2004). Levels of overweight and obesity, defined by Body Mass Index (BMI) are in general increasing across Europe and elsewhere (Lobstein and Frelut, 2003; Wang and Lobstein, 2006). Rates in the UK have risen by almost 400% over 25 years: in England, 23% of men and 25% of women were classified as obese in 2005, with 43% and 34% of men and women respectively overweight (Information Centre for Health and Social Care, 2005). Similarly, in Scotland, 22% of men and 26% of women were obese in 2003, and 65% of men and 60% of women overweight (Scottish Executive, 2005). Nearly two million schoolchildren in the UK are overweight, of whom about 700,000 are obese (Jackson-Leach and Lobstein, 2006), and rates in Scotland are worse than in the rest of the UK.[1]

However, the relationship between rising overweight/obesity levels and socioeconomic status is not simple: the size of differentials depends on which social indicators are used (whether household income, social class, receipt of means-tested benefits or area deprivation scores), and the relationship between socioeconomic conditions of childhood and development of obesity over time is probably important too (Okasha et al, 2003). Nonetheless, there is emerging evidence that income or area deprivation – material circumstances – are critically important. Stamatakis et al (2005) found that household income, rather than a binary occupation-based indicator (manual versus non-manual), predicted childhood obesity; Kinra et al (2000) showed enumeration district deprivation scores were inversely associated with obesity, and independently predicted BMI at age seven years (Kinra et al, 2005).

Kinra's studies, among others, indicate the importance of both household socioeconomic status and the wider social and economic environment for children. A number of studies demonstrate this ecological effect for adults too: obesity measured by BMI was independently related to the degree of income inequality at state level in the US (Diez-Roux et al, 2000), and even at country level (Pickett et al, 2005). Looking specifically at abdominal obesity, which has more profound implications for morbidity and mortality, Ellaway et al (1997) and Kahn et al (1998) found a similar area effect in Scotland and the US respectively: in other words, those living in areas of greater socioeconomic deprivation were not only more likely to gain weight, they were also more likely to gain weight around their middle, particularly men. This effect was independent of other factors such as age, smoking behaviour and individual level deprivation. There are also racial or ethnic differences: in the US, people classified as African American or Hispanic have higher rates of obesity (Kumanyika, 2005), and in the UK, people of South Asian origin tend to have a more central fat distribution.

## Food, nutrition and health

Patterns of food usage and specific nutrient intakes play a critical role in mediating health outcomes (Davey Smith and Brunner, 1997; James et al, 1997; Dowler et al, 2001a; Key et al, 2004), a role that is now more widely recognised in public and policy discourse (Acheson, 1998; WHO/FAO, 2003). The general health benefits of a diet rich in fruits and vegetables (including pulses) have been known for centuries, but now, epidemiological and biochemical evidence has demonstrated that the more fruit and vegetables people eat, the lower their risk of cardiovascular disease (CVD), non-insulin dependent diabetes (NIDDM) and various cancers (Joffe and Robertson, 2001; Pomerleau et al, 2003; WHO/FAO, 2003). Recent calculations in the European Union showed that low fruit and vegetable consumption probably contributed 4.4%, and being overweight or obese added a further 7.8%, to the estimated burden of disease for member states; these two together exceeded the impact of tobacco and alcohol (Pomerleau et al, 2003).

Fruit and vegetable consumption is also a marker for other dietary characteristics thought desirable from a health perspective: those who eat large amounts are also more likely to have high intakes of dietary fibre, low intakes of dietary fats, especially saturated fats, and to eat a varied diet. These patterns are known to reduce disease risk: for instance, about a third of cancers are thought to be diet-related. The epidemiological importance of food intake patterns per se, rather than just individual nutrients, is being increasingly recognised, both because of the biochemical complexity of whole foods and their effects, and the realities of people's responses to health messages (Bazzano, 2005). In epidemiological research, however, indicators of dietary patterns are in fact still fairly crude (Jacques and Tucker, 2001); most surveys simply characterise fruit and vegetable consumption as 'high' or 'low', often in relation to the population mean, and usually find that lower socioeconomic groups are more likely to be in the 'low' group. In practice, though, many populations as a whole consume less fruit and vegetables than thought desirable; it is not only those who are poor who eat insufficient amounts for health.

Obesity also has a direct, independent link to CVD, NIDDM, high blood pressure and some cancers, as well as other conditions such as osteoporosis, particularly where weight gain is abdominal (NAO, 2001; HC, 2004). In the UK, there are now more than two million diabetics (projected to rise to three million by 2010) and there is also increasing insulin resistance, particularly in children, among whom NIDDM is rising (HC, 2004). Obese adults have a nine-year reduction in life expectancy, particularly those with central obesity and/or who also smoke – which is also highly socially patterned (HC, 2004; see also Chapter Nine of this volume). Unsurprisingly, there is also considerable social and psychological stigma to being obese, especially for children. However, the economic implications of obesity are the main reason for current government anxieties. In the UK, in terms of NHS costs and loss of earnings, obesity costs are estimated at between £3.3 and £3.7 billion; if overweight is included, costs are between £6.6 and £7.4 billion (HC, 2004). Of course, these figures do not take into account personal distress from sickness, incapacity, loss of employment and self-esteem, and general misery. Such costs, which are more difficult to estimate, are much more likely to accrue to poorer people.

## Understanding causes and mechanisms

There is a long history of health and other professionals describing the dietary practices of working- or manual-class people as unhealthy or inadequate because of nutritional or housekeeping ignorance or illiteracy, and attributing to them generally undesirable habits (people 'do not spend money wisely and do not know how to shop, budget and cook healthy food'). In part, this practice derives from assumptions that elide 'social class', as representing people's identities, cultural realities and lived, daily experiences, with 'socioeconomic status', representing a statistical grouping of specific measurable indices (Crotty and Germov, 2004, p 244; see also Chapter Four of this volume). These indices include household income, receipt of means-tested benefits, area-level composite deprivation scores, education or occupation – used variously in the studies referred to earlier. They are probably not simply interchangeable in their explanatory power, since their relationship with food–purchasing patterns or nutritional outcomes may differ (Dowler, 2001; Turrell et al, 2002), as the literature briefly cited demonstrates. However, in the absence of fuller models of understanding, indices of socioeconomic well-being are used in epidemiological manipulation of data on measurable 'inputs', 'intermediary determinants' and 'outcomes'; the latter being, in the current instance, nutrient intakes, dietary patterns or obesity.

It is, in fact, quite a challenge to disentangle the relationships between the foods people choose to eat (and why, how, where and with whom they eat them) and their personal social and economic circumstances, as well as the major drivers of food culture and consumption choices in contemporary societies. Figure 8.1, which has been used in various forms for about a decade, is an attempt to map out, from the household perspective, the potential important determinants of what foods are bought and consumed; socioeconomic circumstances at individual, household or area level clearly condition many of these determinants.

Not illustrated but critically shaping and driving food choice are the major trends in the food system: market globalisation with power concentration;[2] increasing availability and promotion of highly processed and ready-prepared foods and meals; state withdrawal from food in social policy, in school meal services and standards and in welfare; loss of local food economies and the increasing dominance of supermarkets; and the growth of food marketing, particularly to children and young people (Nestle, 2002; Lang and Heasman, 2004). Recent work evaluating a decade of Scottish food policy highlighted the difficulty of establishing the role these major trends play in determining food choice; whether they are also exacerbating social and economic inequalities in diet or diminishing them is hotly debated (Lang et al, 2006).

Of course, class, as in cultural or ethnic identity, plays some part in food commodity choices and patterns of using food (Lupton, 1996; Murcott, 2002), but even these differences are becoming harder to characterise consistently as societies become both more eclectic and more homogenous in practice. For instance, some 75% of food sales in the UK are from four major retailers (Tesco, Sainsbury, Asda–Walmart and Morrisons), which also sell increasing amounts of cook-chill 'ready-made' meals: composite dishes that represent a variety of cuisines and tastes. Whether poorer people buy more 'ready meals' than do richer is a moot point; they certainly buy different convenience foods, and may be more likely to buy the familiar, which can be divided into predictable portions. Trying new dishes, particularly those that rely on home cooking where outcomes can be unpredictable, is not a sensible

# Figure 8.1: Determinants of food and nutrition intakes in the UK

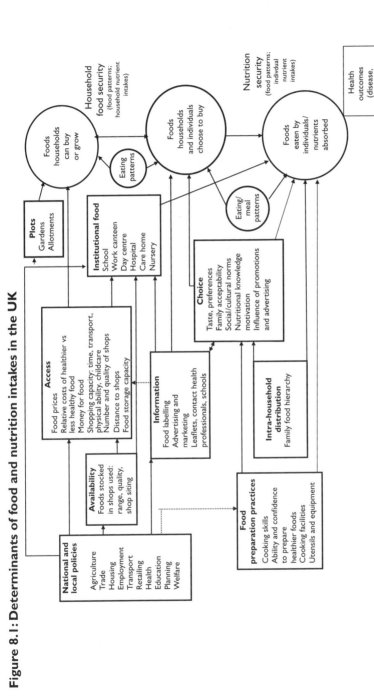

*Source:* Modified from DH (1996) and Dowler et al (2001).

strategy for those on a tight budget with no room for experimentation or failure. Health outcomes such as avoiding heart disease, diabetes, high blood pressure or cancers probably play some part in people's day-to-day food decisions, but in poorer households, particularly those where money is scarce, such considerations may well be less immediate than pleasing the family or friends and being able to eat relatively quickly. There has also been continual anxiety from policy makers and professionals over the loss of cooking skills (Nestle, 2002; Lang and Heasman, 2004, among many); this concern often focuses on the needs of lower socioeconomic groups, whose abilities are thought to be especially important (Wrieden et al, 2007). In fact, the evidence on socioeconomic differentials is equivocal (Caraher et al, 1999) and some dispute whether there has been such a loss of cooking skills, not least because of the difficulties in defining and measuring practice (Short, 2006).

Less tangible are the social norms and expectations of peer groups and society in general, and the factors that shape and change them. The rise in obesity and its potential costs to society have sharpened the debate on the role of TV and other advertising on food purchasing, particularly that geared towards children. Evidence of a damaging effect has recently emerged (Hastings et al, 2003; Ofcom, 2004; Caraher et al, 2006), since many argue that the majority of advertising promotes food that is more likely to be highly processed and unhealthy (EHN, 2005). This in particular is argued to contribute to the general rise in obesity in adults and children, through encouraging increased consumption of energy-dense foods high in saturated fat and sugar, particularly 'fast foods', along with less physical activity and low fruit and vegetable intake (Prentice and Jebb, 2003; Drewnowski and Specter, 2004; Astrup et al, 2006). The social distribution of obesity may also be a product of early life experience compounded by subsequent material and social conditions; hence the importance of a life-course approach and early intervention (National Heart Forum, 2003). Whether poorer people watch more commercial television, are less active, or live where there are more likely to be fast food shops is debatable (Dowler, 2001; Prentice and Jebb, 2003; Cummins and Macintyre, 2005; Sturm and Datar, 2005), but their lower fruit and vegetable intake is a consistent finding (Blanchette and Brug, 2005; Sturm and Datar, 2005). As Lobstein and Frelut put it:

> Poor maternal and foetal nourishment and a low level of breastfeeding may lead to rapid weight gain in an infant's early months, predisposing to shorter stature and central

> adiposity. The dynamics are compounded by a childhood
> diet based on energy-dense foods and a low intake of fruit
> and vegetables, and an urban culture with lower levels of
> physical activity. (Lobstein and Frelut, 2003, p 199)

Much of the research in the 1980s and 1990s on why people on low
incomes or in areas of deprivation bought the food they did pointed to
the importance of material and structural issues of how much money
people had, what food was available and at what cost in the shops that
people used (often subsumed under the term 'access'), as well as skills,
taste and cultural aspects (for example, Caraher et al, 1998). More recent,
questionnaire-based research examining low-income households'
thinking and priorities about food choice has found these latter factors,
along with 'beliefs' (often subsumed under the term 'attitudes') to be
rated by respondents as more important than commodity availability
or physical access to large supermarkets (for instance, Dibsdall et al,
2003; White et al, 2004). These apparent differences may be as much
a reflection of methodology as of a fundamental reality, in that the
characteristics of the physical and social environment in which people
live or work play a critical role in shaping and framing the largely
unconscious, everyday practices of food purchase and consumption,
so that 'availability and access' are not 'perceived', whether the type
and location of shops and markets, or the provision in schools or
workplace canteens.

The Acheson Inquiry, in reflecting the then current research on the
importance of availability, affordability and access, thus departed from
previous explanations for why poor people ate badly that were located
in behaviour and taste. This focus has spawned a research agenda since
the inquiry, in that the UK Economic and Social Research Council
and government have funded retail mapping,[3] and the salience of
the notion of 'food deserts' has been widely debated (Wrigley, 2002).
Cummins and Macintyre (2005) argue that evidence for availability
and price being worse in areas where poorer people live is not found
in Glasgow or Brisbane, and two quasi experimental studies (Wrigley
et al, 2003; Cummins et al, 2005, cited in Cummins and Macintyre,
2005) suggest that access to a reasonable range of cheaper fruit and
vegetables via a new large supermarket does not radically change
purchasing patterns or intakes in low-income households. (However,
this research, unlike that of Morris and his colleagues (2000; 2005) does
not explore the relationship of food prices to actual income, or to that
which is available for food expenditure in the participating households.
Qualitative research in the Glasgow study highlighted local people's

antipathy to the supermarket advent.) White et al (2004), in a detailed study of Newcastle's food shopping, found that retail-related factors were not important predictors of food patterns for the majority of the population, who shopped at larger supermarkets where the range of 'healthier' food, including quality fruit and vegetables, was better than in smaller 'convenience' stores. But there were some areas of the city where it was hard to obtain reasonably priced fresh fruit and vegetables in local shops. This finding is echoed in other studies: Dowler et al (2001b) showed marked variation in availability and price of fruit and vegetables in an area of deprivation in the West Midlands, and others have shown the prices of basic food commodities to be higher in shops where poorer people live than in large supermarkets, which are often located for car users (as was the case in White et al, 2004).

For those on low incomes, where basic expenditures such as rent, fuel and water absorb a high proportion of outgoings – costs that have risen faster than the retail price index in recent years, and may vary around the country, unlike income from benefits, pensions or the minimum wage – the cost of food relative to other essentials can be very critical in determining purchasing patterns (Dowler, 2003). Households may have very little flexibility in how they prioritise expenditures: compulsory deductions of arrears, or fines (or worse) for defaulting on paying bills or rent, mean that food often represents the only flexible budget item (Dobson et al, 1994; Dowler et al, 2001a). Qualitative research shows that people economise either by buying cheaper or different items (no fruit, fewer vegetables, cheap processed meats, filling instant foods), or by omitting meals altogether (relying on sandwiches, breakfast cereals, or nothing). Over the past two decades, the poorest communities have also faced multiple deprivations of unemployment and inadequate housing, despite regeneration initiatives, along with the withdrawal of basic services and amenities such as banks and food retailers. Travel costs to reach supermarkets (where prices may be lower than local shops) can mean economising on 'luxury' items such as fruit.

In the UK, the term 'food poverty' has increasingly been used by academics and policy makers to describe these circumstances: where households or individuals are 'unable to acquire or consume adequate quality or sufficient quantity of food in socially acceptable ways, or the uncertainty that one will be able to do so' (Riches, 1996, cited in Dowler et al, 2001a, p 2). The assumption is that material conditions rather than intransigence are key. Few studies to date have been able to differentiate short- and long-term impacts of low incomes or living in areas of deprivation on food patterns and nutrient intakes. The Department for Work and Pensions is attempting to monitor long-term poverty and its effects, and the forthcoming Food Standards Agency-funded survey should provide useful data. Research using a budget standards approach has demonstrated that UK families with dependent children (Parker et al, 1998), young single men paid at or below the minimum wage (Morris et al, 2000) and older people living on state pensions (Morris et al, 2005) have insufficient money to meet basic needs for healthy living.

The definition of food poverty also recognises social acceptability: food as an expression of identity and ability to provide for the family – issues not readily assessed in epidemiological surveys or national surveillance. If you have to eat in a day centre[4] or shop in an unappealing discount store, or if your local shops are inadequately stocked with poor-quality or more expensive food, or your children cannot have a packed lunch similar to that of their friends, you are not living in ways deemed normal by the rest of society, whatever your nutrient intake. In the Republic of Ireland the National Anti-Poverty Strategy uses some normative expectations of foods and meals (rather than nutrients) as part of its measure of 'consistent' poverty,[5] combining a relative income measure with a composite deprivation index of eight items, three of which relate to food: having a meal with meat, fish or chicken every second day; having a roast or its equivalent once a week; not having gone without a substantial meal in the last two weeks. These indices are similar to the consensually defined necessities of the Poverty and Social Exclusion Surveys (discussed in Dowler, 2003). People do not have to use or consume these things, but they should be able to do so – they should have the resources (money, time) and access to express normative choices. Whether or not the term 'food poverty' is used, the fact that there are people living in material circumstances that make it very difficult to purchase or obtain the food they need for healthy living is an important one, and potentially sidesteps debates about whether or not people *choose* to eat in ways that are not conducive to health, in the shorter and longer term.

There has been a growth in use of participative research methods, particularly by local authorities and civil society, which gives voice to the wider perceptions of those living in conditions of deprivation, both in analysing the problem and pointing to solutions. These methods also enable the particular combinations of factors in a given place or set of social circumstances to be established and inform local response, particularly to inequalities.[6] Such approaches may be of variable quality, but they can also sometimes be very creative in methodological approach and intersectoral involvement (Johnson and Webster, 2000).

## Policy responses to food and nutrition inequalities in the UK

Inequalities in food and nutritional status have long been acknowledged in the UK, although contributory factors have mostly been seen as an aspect of 'lifestyle' – a failing in household management and individual choice. The alternative has also been argued, that nutritional inequalities represent the outcome of a set of structural problems: individuals or households lack access to or control over resources, or opportunities to secure a reasonable livelihood; they live (or work) in places where food conducive to health is not readily available at affordable prices, but where cheap, filling food that does not confirm to nutritional guidelines for health is widely available; they are bombarded with advertising for the latter rather than the former. As a result, they find it very difficult to adopt a healthy diet. These distinctions are crucial for policy response. If 'lifestyle choices' are at fault, the role of the state at national or local level is to offer corrective information and skills delivery to enable appropriate choice, and market liberalisation to allow such choice efficient expression. Where people make 'wrong choices', better ways of providing information and/or skills is needed. If structural problems are key, the state's responsibility is one of regulating access to and control over food (including the role of multinationals in food procurement and distribution) and other resources, such as jobs, wages and income levels. The Acheson Inquiry largely took the second view: that structural issues of access and income levels were crucial to reducing inequalities in food and nutrition. However, despite some promising early initiatives, such as free fruit in schools and the introduction of a minimum wage, much of the intervention since has focused on local projects and promotional schemes, characterised by downstream, modest short-term investments. The drift back to 'lifestyle choices' is all too apparent (see also Chapters Three and Four for discussion of this drift).

The Acheson Inquiry built on several years' work by civil society campaigning and advocacy groups and some academic research, as well as the work of a small Low Income and Diet Project Team (under the previous Conservative government's Nutrition Task Force) (Leather, 1996; Dowler et al, 2001a). The report of this project team, despite a remit to identify examples of good practice in local initiatives and projects, had addressed structural and material issues as well, such as changes in food retailing (but not the adequacy of benefit levels, which was specifically excluded; see Leather, 1992), and the responsibilities of local and national government (DH, 1996). It called for a national

network of local initiatives on food and low income, and the creation
of local public/private sector food partnerships, especially in areas of
multiple disadvantage, to regenerate local food economies. The former
happened under the aegis of Sustain's Food Poverty project[7] and the
latter has slowly developed in one or two places.[8] As it happened,
Acheson himself chaired one of the meetings promoting the project
team's recommendations, held within weeks of the Labour election
landslide in May 1997, at which the then new Secretary of State for
Public Health, Tessa Jowell, was present. Perhaps as a result, food access
was mentioned as an issue in the early public health White Paper
(DH, 1999a); it was certainly highlighted in the Acheson Report
(Acheson, 1998), along with two other national level issues, in its
recommendations:

- increase availability and accessibility of an adequate and affordable
  diet, and specifically policies to ensure adequate retail provision of
  food to those who are disadvantaged;
- review the Common Agricultural Policy (CAP)'s impact on
  inequalities in health;
- strengthen the CAP Surplus Food Scheme to improve the
  nutritional position of the less well off.

Other indirect food recommendations referred to social security
benefits, transport and breastfeeding (the latter is addressed in Chapter
Five).

There was no coordinated policy response to nutrition and food
inequalities. The newly created Social Exclusion Unit (SEU) reported
on problems in the retail sector in deprived areas in a consultation
document that contained useful recommendations about community-
based retailing and small businesses strategies (DH, 1999b). However,
little central government activity followed, and no mechanism was
ever set up to coordinate activity. A subsequent SEU report (2001) set
quantified targets for improving the most deprived neighbourhoods in
England (with similar publications for Scotland and Wales), but access
to shops or appropriate food had largely disappeared from the national
regeneration agenda. As mentioned earlier, there has been investment in
research on physical and, to some extent, economic, access to healthy
food, particularly fresh fruit and vegetables; the equivocal results seem
not to have engendered government response. There were some
elements of addressing access in the Department of Health's 'Five a
Day' programme, but this was probably more a result of the approach
of professionals on the ground than any policy to improve access. There

have been a few initiatives on social and retail planning, and rather more on attempting to change consumer demand, so that, for instance, local shops where poorer people live will stock 'healthier' food ranges in response (Caraher, 2005). More effective public health solutions probably lie in addressing the 'upstream' structural issues, rather than in trying to influence individual 'attitudes'. There are few nutrition policies that explicitly address reduction of inequalities (this issue is discussed in Lang et al, 2006); more usually, interventions have simply been targeted at areas of deprivation, in the hope that this will capture low socioeconomic household groups and improve their nutritional circumstances. The effectiveness and merits of a universalist, population approach, as opposed to a selectivist or targeted one, to meet the needs of particular groups is debated in the public health literature, and some of the issues apply when targeting is by socioeconomic status (Prättälä et al, 2002).

The Acheson Inquiry was concerned with England and Wales; in Scotland, the adoption of the Scottish Diet Action Plan in 1996 built on a clear statement of inequalities in outcomes reflecting unequal access, availability and behavioural demand (Scottish Office, 1994). There was a call to remove 'barriers' to healthy eating for people on low incomes. In practice, as a recent evaluation has shown, there has been no reduction in nutritional inequalities (and in fact no improvement in average intakes); the reasons for such a policy failure are complex but include a loss of focus, which permitted too many disparate initiatives (Lang et al, 2006). In Wales, an initiative on food and well-being was launched in 2003; this also included statements about access and the need to address the role of the food industry (FSAW, 2003). Most activity to date has been project-based; a mid-term evaluation is currently under way.

The 'School Fruit Scheme' was gradually rolled out across England, with a parallel scheme in Scotland, and entitled all four- to six-year-old children in local education authority-maintained infant, primary and special schools to a free piece of fruit (and now vegetables) each school day because 'for too many families, access to healthy food is limited, especially in some low income areas where affordable fruit and vegetables can be hard to find' (DH, 2002, p 1). Early evaluation has emphasised successes in terms of process and results.[9] School breakfast initiatives in England, Scotland and Wales have also been promoted and partially funded by central government, at least initially, some of which were framed in terms of access problems, although probably more from recognition of household or parental failure to provide food early in the day. Free fruit and vegetable schemes are now funded from the New Opportunities Fund, the largest of the lottery good cause distributors.

A main focus for government activity has been the development of a wide range of local food initiatives and projects, which sometimes give immediate, short-term benefits but often fail to address fundamental issues (Dowler and Caraher, 2003) and which lack a comprehensive, competent strategic base. From 2000, government national responses to nutrition inequalities coalesced in the health sector around the 'Five a Day'[10] (fruit and vegetable) programme and the National School Fruit Scheme (DH, 2002). However, despite the rhetoric, one could argue that both were designed more to address general low fruit and vegetable intakes rather than inequalities. The community-based 'Five a Day' work was largely project-structured and was generally located in areas of deprivation, but whether the benefits significantly accrued to poorer households and their members is questionable. There is also evidence that as the current policy agenda has switched to addressing obesity, particularly in children, continual support for fruit and vegetable promotion is less secure. The inequalities dimension to obesity is acknowledged but not often explicitly addressed except under individual aspects of 'lifestyle'.

Most projects, rather than tackling the determinants of inequalities, focus on skills of cooking, household management or, occasionally, growing (McGlone et al, 1999; Caraher and Dowler, 2007). There has been a great fashion for 'food cooperatives' to address 'access' issues, but encouraging people who live on very low incomes, who are often time poor (for example, because they are lone parents) or unskilled, to source fresh produce locally and then manage distribution and recovery of financial outlay through volunteer systems is hardly a plausible sustainable solution to the fundamental challenges of contemporary food retailing and local regeneration.[11] Indeed, some argue that regeneration in practice now more often means support for fast food outlets, 'gastro-pubs' and gambling. The emphasis could thus be seen as helping those who are poor to help themselves to tackle the inequalities that professionals find challenging. Of course, there are some good local examples of imaginative, coordinated activities that build on local people's identification of needs and where solutions attempt to address both structural issues and personal skills and the desire for celebration of food cultures, but these are rare in a field where projects come and go with funding and the current policy agenda.

Those working on local projects in fact often struggle with a shifting policy context for their work: NHS reforms, National Service Frameworks for prevention and care, the National Cancer Plan, and health inequalities, many of which focus more on secondary than primary prevention. The recent location of decision making and money at local level (through Primary Care Trusts and local authority structures such as Local Strategic Partnerships and Local Area Agreements) means that food and community development can lose out to government 'must do' acute service priorities such as reducing waiting lists (Caraher and Dowler, 2007), not least because the food projects lack designated funding. The UK Chief Medical Officer warned of the diversion of public health budgets to clinical targets, with concomitant loss of small-scale local projects and their skills, in his 2006 report (DH, 2006). Targeting by deprivation area is a common practice (see Chapter Eleven of this volume), but implementation has been patchy, not well supported and left to a mix of local funding mechanisms, which means many ground-level staff operate on short contracts. Furthermore, not all people on lower incomes live in areas of deprivation (Joshi et al, 2000). A major funding source in the late 1990s and early 2000s was the Community Fund, sourced from the National Lottery; the Big Lottery Fund was formed from the merger of the Community Fund and the New Opportunities Fund. It currently distributes around £600 million annually (half the 'good cause' funding from the National Lottery). The Big Lottery Fund is now a major player in funding health, education and environmental projects, with emphasis on tackling disadvantage and working through voluntary groups supporting community improvement. This arguably represents a move from state welfare funding as part of a public health agenda to one based on charity and a philosophical move from rights to benevolence.

Reform of the Welfare Food Scheme to re-emerge as Healthy Start in 2004 has switched a food-related income transfer programme into a potentially more restrictive nutrition intervention programme, and subsumed welfare under the Department of Health, with links into Sure Start local programmes and now Children's Centres. School meals have also been a growing focus for anxieties and somewhat piecemeal solutions (Gustafsson, 2002). The recent government attention to school meal quality, sourcing and quantity has little explicit focus on inequalities (Morgan, 2006). Indeed, the likelihood is that parental costs will increase with quality improvement, which will make further demands on low-income households. The eligibility for free school meals has narrowed and become more complicated with the advent of child tax credit; many children who live in poor households do not qualify, and 25% of those who are eligible fail to claim because of stigma and other reasons (Dowler et al, 2001a; Riley, 2005). Again, there is a shifting of responsibility for feeding poorer children from the state to low-income parents, who usually have little control over what is offered, at what price and under what circumstances, in schools. The result is often that children bring unhealthy packed lunches or spend their limited 'dinner money' on cheap fast foods such as chips, which are often readily available just outside the school gates. Campaigns for universal free primary school meals, such as that in Scotland, can draw on the example of Hull City Council, where school meal take-up doubled over two years and pupil learning capacity improved as a result of healthier intakes.[12]

The CAP's impact on health and nutrition has largely been addressed by European alliances (for example, Schäfer Elinder et al, 2003; Robertson et al, 2004) and civil society organisations (for example, Sustain and the UK Food Group, 2002) that work hard to keep public health on the discussions agenda, with some academic research support. However, the current discussions on CAP reform do not start until 2008, with implementation in 2013, and the key UK government document (HM Treasury and Defra, 2005) makes no mention of health at all, let alone inequalities. The UK lead on health inequalities during its 2005 presidency of the EU raised salient issues including the role of diet.[13] In 2006, the EU produced a Green Paper on nutrition, building on work from a forum of partners including the food and marketing industries and civil society groups (such as the National Heart Forum), some of whom focus on inequalities issues. There has been scope for comment on structural issues as well as on addressing the 'clustering of unhealthy habits' (EU Commission, 2005, p 10).

The effects of the CAP Surplus Food Scheme are poorly understood and publicised (Lang, 2002; Sustain and the UK Food Group, 2002). One long-criticised effect of the CAP is overproduction of subsidised foods; the scheme redistributes easily stored foods (such as butter, canned meat) to those who are less well off, but does not cover fresh produce such as fruit and vegetables, whose surpluses are routinely destroyed (Lobstein and Longfield, 1999; Robertson et al, 2004). The subsidies also, it is argued, maintain food prices higher than they need be, which affects poorer people more than richer, since the former spend a higher proportion of their income on food.

## Present and future realities?

Two major reviews by Wanless (2002, 2004) for the Treasury of the social and economic costs of ignoring the health impact of current trends were significant for their espousal of the role of food and nutrition in contributing to health inequalities. Problem statements from the late

1990s therefore gained a degree of credibility and urgency, but the challenges remain the identification, establishment and coordination of appropriate policy response, and recognising 'food' within the experience and definitions of poverty. The 2004 England White Paper *Choosing health: Making healthier choices easier* (DH, 2004) in pushing an individualisation agenda for food relegated the state's role, apart from the residual responsibility for welfare food provision, to one of changing individual perceptions and practice so people assume more responsibility for their own lifestyles and thus food choice. The White Paper signalled powerful potential policy shifts, towards social marketing and partnership working with the food and marketing industries in particular, whose impact on inequalities is very unclear. The source of sufficient, appropriate funding is critical, as will be the 'upstream: downstream' balance of policy focus. Will 'poor food' still turn out to be 'poor people's' responsibility (Food Ethics Council, 2005)?

Interest in public health nutrition across government has been galvanised by the potential costs of the obesity 'crisis',[14] but the extent to which obesity will derail the wider agenda, and particularly attempts to address inequalities, is unclear. The recent DH food and health action plan (2005), however, potentially represents a competent policy framework and has an upstream systematic strategy for improving public health nutrition in England, although it has no explicit inequalities focus. The Scottish Executive's acceptance of the upstream, structural recommendations, including the need to build inequalities into targets, in the recent report evaluating a decade of nutrition policy, is similarly promising (Lang et al, 2006), although in neither country are signals always translated into coherent policy activity. The food and health plan includes a comprehensive approach to reshaping the food economy and culture through social marketing, front-of-pack 'consumer-friendly' food labelling, restrictions on food marketing to children, encouraging processed food reformulation, school meal standards, public food procurement and moves to reform the CAP on a health agenda.

The food and health plan has yet to be fully funded and implemented, and the extent to which government will regulate the food and marketing industries and champion these issues in Europe is unknown. The Food Standards Agency was charged with leading on food labelling, food marketing to children and food reformulation, starting with salt reductions. Despite some successes, its experience with supporting research on clearer product labelling, for instance, has been mixed: consumer and public interest groups favour a colour-coded 'traffic-light' system, whereas some key food companies reject it as too simple.[15] The UK government has not yet regulated labelling (an EU competency) but may push to do so; it has recently announced regulation of TV marketing of foods high in fat, sugar and salt, particularly to children (a 9pm food marketing watershed is still under debate). But the food and health plan is a whole-population approach; the possibilities for reducing nutrition and health inequalities is unclear, not least since there are few good practice examples of government addressing structural issues to reduce food inequalities. Public procurement for school meals led by Scotland and Wales are important potential models and drivers for change.

## Conclusion

This chapter has outlined the continuing inequalities in food patterns and nutrient intakes in the UK, and summarised current research that contributes to understanding why these inequalities persist. Space has precluded discussion of the wider environmental challenges of retail and planning demands, the impacts of food system globalisation (both on commodity availability and cost, and on advertising) and regulatory mechanisms at national, regional and global levels (see Nestle, 2002; Lang and Heasman, 2004; Lang et al, 2006). The response by government at national level has tended to focus on 'lifestyle' changes, using the model of a responsibility partnership between the state and individuals: that people should be facilitated to choose food that contributes to their health. However, for many people, choice is proscribed by factors outside their control. Furthermore, attempts to change deeply imbedded social behavioural patterns by using the negative language of 'barriers', which often reinforces hierarchical social distinctions of 'taste', are less likely to succeed than those that embrace people's own aspirations and desires, and actively engage in enabling their achievement.

Serious response to the structural dimensions of the food system that are beyond consumer control at national government level was mooted in the late 1990s and features to some extent in the 2005 food and health action plan. 'Food labelling', partial response to the 1980s privatisation of school food provision, and recent restrictions on TV advertising are evidence of the beginnings of an engagement at population level to change food culture and economy, but the food industry is largely seen as a benign partner rather than having responsibility for causing as well as curing the problem, particularly in England. Increasingly, the state actively engages with the food industry, in its widest aspects, to achieve 'better behaviour', particularly among those on low incomes. The extent to which the current raft of changes will address health inequalities in food and nutrition is unknown and as yet unmonitored. More imaginative approaches have been taken at local authority level to try to reduce the constraints of availability and affordability for good food for all; but even these have yet to be mainstreamed or shown to make substantial, measurable difference to food outcomes.

The food civil society lobby in the UK has grown in strength and effectiveness, contributing to raising issues about rights and entitlement to food (Riches, 2003) as a public health good, instead of merely a focus for benevolence or private activity as a 'lifestyle' choice. Tackling inequalities in food and nutrition requires serious 'upstream' intervention, but the complexities of both the food system and people's engagement with it (simplified in Figure 8.1) require imaginative and courageous cross-sectoral working. Only thus can all citizens – and those without even that label and associated rights – be enabled to enjoy food conducive to healthy living in all its aspects.

**Notes**

[1] Scottish Health Statistics: website of Information and Statistics Division (ISD) Scotland (www.isdscotland.org/isd/info3.jsp?pContentID= 3640&p_applic=CCC&p_service=Content.show&).

[2] See Food Ethics Council publications May-July 2005: 'Power in the food system' (www.foodethicscouncil.org/node/103).

[3] For example, the Food Standards Agency commissioned White et al (2004) to examine the realities of 'food deserts' in Newcastle, and the Food Standards Agency Scotland commissioned Dawson et al (www. csrs.ac.uk/fsa.htm) to map food access throughout Scotland (J. Dawson, M. Taylor, D. Marshall, L. Sparks, S. Cummins and A. Anderson, 'Accessing healthy food: a national assessment and sentinel mapping study of food retailing in Scotland'). The Department of Health has also funded 'food access' work.

[4] In 2005, 2,000 tonnes of food was redistributed through a community food network of 300 organisations to 12,000 disadvantaged people each day in 34 cities and towns across the UK (http://fareshare.org. uk/about/index.html).

[5] www.socialinclusion.ie/poverty.html

[6] For examples, see Sustain Food Access Network (formerly food poverty) database (www.sustainweb.org); Community Food and Health (Scotland) (formerly Scottish Community Diet Project) (www. communityfoodandhealth.org.uk); Nutrition Network Wales (www. nutritionnetworkwales.org.uk).

[7] Now Food Access Network (www.sustainweb.org/page.php?id=50).

[8] For example, Sandwell West Midlands food policy (www.rrt-pct.org. uk/healthy_living/food-policy.htm); Greenwich food policy (www. greenwich.gov.uk/Greenwich/CommunityLiving/HealthFood/ FoodNutrition/FoodPolicy.htm); Brighton and Hove food strategy (www.bhfood.org.uk).

[9] For England, see www.nfer.ac.uk/research-areas/pims-data/outlines/ further-evaluation-of-the-school.cfm; for Scotland, www.scotland.gov. uk/Publications/2005/12/21110322/03222; for Northern Ireland, www.investingforhealthni.gov.uk/fruit.asp

[10] www.5aday.nhs.uk and www.dh.gov.uk/PolicyAndGuidance/ HealthAndSocialCareTopics/FiveADay/fs/en

[11] At the time of writing, a third Competition Commission Inquiry into the grocery market is under way.

[12] At the time of writing, Hull City Council has reversed a recent decision to stop funding free universal primary school meals until the end of the summer term in 2007, but made the continual funding an issue in the May council elections (http://education.guardian.co.uk/ schoolmeals/story/0,,2025227,00.html).

[13] www.dh.gov.uk/PolicyAndGuidance/International/EuropeanUnion/ EUPresidency2005/fs/en; follow the links to Tackling Inequalities in Health programme.

[14] For instance, the Department of Trade and Industry has commissioned Foresight to look more closely at the possible consequences of the obesity epidemic over the next 50 years.

[15] www.eatwell.gov.uk/foodlabels/trafficlights

## References

Acheson, D. (1998) *Independent inquiry into inequalities in health*, London: The Stationery Office.

Astrup, A., Bovy, M.W.L., Nackenhors, K. and Popova, A.E. (2006) 'Food for thought or thought for food? A stakeholder dialogue around the role of the snacking industry in addressing the obesity epidemic', *Obesity Reviews*, vol 7, no 3, pp 303-12.

Bazzano, L.A. (2005) 'Dietary intake of fruit and vegetables and risk of diabetes mellitus and cardiovascular diseases', Background paper for joint Food and Agriculture Organisation/World Health Organization Workshop on Fruit and Vegetables for Health, Japan.

Blanchette, L. and Brug, J. (2005) 'Determinants of fruit and vegetable consumption among 6-12-year-old children and effective interventions to increase consumption', *Journal of Human Nutrition and Dietetics*, vol 18, no 6, pp 431-43.

Caraher, M. (2005) 'Food policy and regeneration: food for thought', *Local Work: Voice. Centre for Local Economic Strategies*, vol 64, pp 1-4.

Caraher, M. and Dowler, E. (2007) 'Food projects in London: lessons for policy and practice', *Health Education Journal*, vol 66, no 2, pp 188-205.

Caraher, M., Dixon, P., Lang, T. and Carr-Hill, R. (1998) 'Barriers to accessing healthy foods: differentials by gender, social class, income and mode of transport', *Health Education Journal*, vol 57, no 3, pp 191-201.

Caraher, M., Landon, J. and Dalmeny, K. (2006) 'Television advertising and children: lessons from policy development', *Public Health Nutrition*, vol 9, no 5, pp 596-605.

Caraher, M., Lang, T., Dixon, P. and Carr-Hill, R. (1999) 'The state of cooking in England: the relationship of cooking skills to food choice', *British Food Journal*, vol 101, no 8, pp 590-609.

Christie, I., Harrison, M., Hitchman, C. and Lang, T. (2002) *Inconvenience food – the struggle to eat well on a low income*, London: Demos.

Crotty, P. and Germov, J. (2004) 'Food and class', in J. Germov and L. Williams (eds) *A sociology of food and nutrition: The social appetite* (2nd edn), Victoria: Oxford University Press, pp 241-62.

Cummins, S. and Macintyre, S. (2005) 'Food environments and obesity – neighbourhood or nation?', *International Journal of Epidemiology*, vol 35, no 1, pp 100-4.

Cummins, S., Petticrew, M., Higgins, C., Findlay, A., Sparks, L. (2005). 'Large scale food retailing as health intervention: quasi-experimental evaluation of a natural experiment', *Journal of Epidemiology and Community Health*, vol 59, no 12, pp 1035-40.

Davey Smith, G. and Brunner, E. (1997) 'Socio-economic differentials in health: the role of nutrition', *Proceedings of the Nutrition Society*, vol 56, no 1A, pp 75-90.

Defra (Department of Food, Environment and Rural Affairs) (2006) *Family food: Report on the Expenditure & Food Survey*, London: Defra (http://statistics.defra.gov.uk/esg/publications/efs/default.asp).

DH (Department of Health) (1996) *Low income, food, nutrition and health: Strategies for improvement*, Report from the Low Income Project Team to the Nutrition Task Force, London: DH.

DH (1999a) *Saving lives: Our healthier nation*, Cm 4386, London: The Stationery Office.

DH (1999b) *Improving shopping access*, Policy Action Team 13, London: DH.

DH (2002) *The National School Fruit Scheme*, London: DH.

DH (2004) *Choosing health: Making healthier choices easier*, Cm 6374, London: The Stationery Office.

DH (2005) *Choosing a better diet: A food and health action plan*, London: DH.

DH (2006) *On the state of the public health: Annual report of the Chief Medical Officer 2005*, London: DH.

Dibsdall, L.A., Lambert, N., Bobbin, R.F. and Frewer, L.J. (2003) 'Low income consumers' attitudes and behaviours towards access, affordability and motivation to eat fruit and vegetables', *Public Health Nutrition*, vol 6, no 2, pp 159-68.

Diez-Roux, A.V., Link, B.G. and Northridge, M.E. (2000) 'A multilevel analysis of income inequality and cardiavascular disease risk factors', *Social Science and Medicine*, vol 50, no 5, pp 673-87.

Dobson, B., Beardsworth, A., Keil, T. and Walker, R. (1994) *Diet, choice and poverty: Social, cultural and nutritional aspects of food consumption among low income families*, London: Family Policy Studies Centre for the Joseph Rowntree Foundation.

Dowler, E. (2001) 'Inequalities in diet and physical activity in Europe', *Public Health Nutrition*, vol 4, no 2B, pp 701-9.

Dowler, E. (2003) 'Food and poverty in Britain: rights and responsibilities', in E. Dowler and C. Jones Finer (eds) *The welfare of food: Rights and responsibilities in a changing world*, Oxford: Blackwell Publishing, pp 140-59.

Dowler, E. and Caraher, M. (2003) 'Local food projects: the new philanthropy?', *Political Quarterly*, vol 74, no 1, pp 57-65.

Dowler, E. and Turner, S. with Dobson, B. (2001a) *Poverty bites: Food, health and poor families*, London: Child Poverty Action Group.

Dowler, E., Blair, A., Rex, D., Donkin, A. and Grundy, C. (2001b) *Mapping access to healthy food in Sandwell*, Report to the Health Action Zone (www.rrt-pct.org.uk/healthy_living/SANDWELL.PDF).

Drewnowski, A. and Specter, S.E. (2004) 'Poverty and obesity: the role of energy density and energy costs', *American Journal of Clinical Nutrition*, vol 79, no 1, pp 6-16.

EHN (European Heart Network) (2005) 'The marketing of unhealthy food to children in Europe' (www.ehnheart.org or www.heartforum. org.uk).

EU Commission (2005) *Promoting healthy diets and physical activity: a European dimension for the prevention of overweight, obesity and chronic diseases*, Green Paper.

Ellaway, A., Anderson, A. and Macintyre, S. (1997) 'Does area of residence affect body size and shape?', *International Journal of Obesity*, vol 21, no 4, pp 304-8.

Finch, S. (1998) *National Diet and Nutrition Survey: People aged 65 years and over. Vol 1: Report of the Diet and Nutrition Survey*, London: The Stationery Office.

Food Ethics Council (2005) *Getting personal: shifting responsibilities for dietary health*, Brighton: Food Ethics Council (http://foodethicscouncil. org/).

FSAW (Food Standards Agency Wales) (2003) *Food and well being: Reducing inequalities through a nutrition strategy for Wales*, Cardiff: Food Standards Agency.

Gregory, J.R. (2000) *National Diet and Nutrition Survey: Young people aged 4–18 years. Vol 1: Report of the Diet and Nutrition Survey*, London: The Stationery Office.

Gregory J.R., Collins, D.L., Davies, P.S.W., Hughes, J.M. and Clarke, P. (1995) *National Diet and Nutrition Survey: Children aged 1.5 to 4.5 years*, London: HMSO.

Gustafsson, U. (2002) 'School meals policy: the problem with governing children', *Social Policy and Administration*, vol 36, no 6, pp 685-97.

Hastings, G., Stead, M., McDermott, L., Forsyth, A., Mackintosh, A.M., Rayner, M., Godfrey, C., Caraher, M. and Angus, K. (2003) *Review of research on the effects of food promotion to children*, Report prepared for the Food Standards Agency, Glasgow: Centre for Social Marketing.

HC (House of Commons Health Committee) (2004) *Obesity. Third report of Session 2003–4. Volume 1*, HC 23-1, London: The Stationery Office.

HM Treasury and Defra (Department for Environment, Food and Rural Affairs) (2005) *A vision for Common Agricultural Policy*, London: The Stationery Office.

Hoare, J., Henderson, L., with Bates, C.J., Prentice, A., Birch, M., Swan, G. and Farron, M. (2004) *National Diet and Nutrition Survey: Adults aged 19 to 64 years. Vol 5: Summary report*, London: The Stationery Office.

Information Centre for Health and Social Care (2006) *Health Survey for England 2005: Updating of trend tables to include 2005 data*, London: The Information Centre for Health and Social Care (www.ic.nhs. uk/pubs/hseupdate05).

Jackson-Leach, R. and Lobstein, T. (2006) 'Estimated burden of paediatric obesity and co-morbidities in Europe. Part 1: The increase in the prevalence of child obesity in Europe is itself increasing', *International Journal of Pediatric Obesity*, vol 1, no 1, pp 26-32.

Jacques, P.F. and Tucker, K.L. (2001) 'Are dietary patterns useful for understanding the role of diet in chronic disease?', *American Journal of Clinical Nutrition*, vol 73, no 1, pp 1-2.

James, W.P.T., Nelson, M., Ralph, A. and Leather, S. (1997) 'Socioeconomic determinants of health: the contribution of nutrition to inequalities in health', *British Medical Journal*, vol 314, pp 1545-9.

Joffe, M. and Robertson, A. (2001) 'The potential contribution of increased vegetable and fruit consumption to health gain in the European Union', *Public Health Nutrition*, vol 4, no 4, pp 893-901.

Johnson, V. and Webster, J. (2000) *'Reaching the parts ...'. Community mapping: Working together to tackle social exclusion and food poverty*, London: Sustain: the Alliance for Better Food and Farming.

Joshi, H., Wiggins, R.D., Bartley, M., Mitchell, R., Gleave, S. and Lynch, K. (2000) 'Putting health inequalities on the map: does where you live matter, and why?' in H. Graham (ed) *Understanding health inequalities*, Buckingham: Open University Press, pp 143-55.

Kahn, H.S., Tatham, L.M., Pamuk, E.R. and Heath, C.W.Jr. (1998) 'Are geographic regions with high income inequality associated with risk of abdominal weight gain?', *Social Science and Medicine*, vol 47, no 1, pp 1-6.

Key, T.J., Schatzkin, A., Willett, W.C., Allen, N.E., Spencer, E.A. and Travis, R.C. (2004) 'Diet, nutrition and the prevention of cancer', *Public Health Nutrition*, vol 7, no 1A, pp 187-200.

Kinra, S., Baumer, J.H. and Davey Smith, G. (2005) 'Early growth and childhood obesity: a historical cohort study', *Archives of Disease in Childhood*, vol 90, no 11, pp 1122-7.

Kinra, S., Nelder, R.P. and Lewendon, G.J. (2000) 'Deprivation and childhood obesity: a cross sectional study of 20,973 children in Plymouth, United Kingdom', *Journal of Epidemiology and Community Health*, vol 54, no 6, pp 456-60.

Kumanyika, S. (2005) 'Obesity, health disparities and prevention paradigms: hard questions and hard choices', *Preventing Chronic Disease*, vol 2 no 4, Epub 15 September (public domain journal online at www.cdc.gov/pcd, accessed 21 August 2006).

Lang, T. (2002) 'Making healthy food a factor in CAP reform', *European Public Health Alliance Food and Agriculture Update 63* (www.epha.org/r/17, accessed 21 August 2006).

Lang, T. and Heasman, M. (2004) *Food wars*, London: Earthscan.

Lang, T., Dowler, E. and Hunter, D. (2006) *Review of the Scottish Diet Action Plan: Progress and impacts 1996–2005*, Edinburgh: NHS Health Scotland (www.healthscotland.com/understanding/evaluation/policy-reviews/review-diet-action.aspx).

Leather, S. (1992) 'Less money, less choice: poverty and diet in the UK today', in National Consumer Council (ed) *Your food: Whose choice?*, London: HMSO, pp 72-94.

Leather, S. (1996) *The making of modern malnutrition: An overview of food poverty in the UK*, London: The Caroline Walker Trust.

Lobstein, T. and Frelut, M.-L. (2003) 'Prevalence of overweight among children in Europe', *Obesity Reviews*, vol 4, no 4, pp 195-200.

Lobstein, T. and Longfield, J. (1999) *Improving diet and health through European Union food policies*, London: Health Education Authority.

Lupton, D. (1996) *Food, the body and the self*, London: Sage Publications.

McGlone, P., Dobson, B., Dowler, E. and Nelson, M. (1999) *Food projects and how they work*, York: York Publishing, for the Joseph Rowntree Foundation.

Morgan, K. (2006) 'School food and the public domain: the politics of the public plate', *Political Quarterly*, vol 77, no 3, pp 379-87.

Morris, J., Dangour, A., Deeming, C., Fletcher, A. and Wilkinson, P. (2005) *Minimum income for healthy living: Older people*, London: Age Concern England.

Morris, J., Donkin, A., Wonderling, D., Wilkinson, P. and Dowler, E. (2000) 'A minimum income for healthy living', *Journal of Epidemiology and Community Health*, vol 54, no 12, pp 885-9.

Murcott, A. (2002) 'Nutrition and inequalities: a note on sociological approaches', *European Journal of Public Health*, vol 12, no 3, pp 203-7.

NAO (National Audit Office) (2001) *Tackling obesity in England*, HC 220, London: The Stationery Office.

National Heart Forum (2003) *A lifecourse approach to coronary heart disease prevention: Scientific and policy review*, London: National Heart Forum.

Nestle, M. (2002) *Food politics: How the food industry influences nutrition and health*, Berkeley, CA: University of California Press.

Ofcom (2004) 'Childhood obesity – food advertising in context: children's food choices, parents' understanding and influence, and the role of food promotion' (www.ofcom.org.uk/research/tv/reports/food_ads).

Okasha, M., McCarron, P., McEwen, J., Durnin, J. and Davey Smith, G. (2003) 'Childhood social class and adulthood obesity: findings from the Glasgow Alumni Cohort', *Journal of Epidemiology and Community Health*, vol 57, no 7, pp 508-9.

Parker, H. with Nelson, M., Oldfield, N., Dallison, J., Hutton, S., Paterakis, S., Sutherland, H. and Thirlwart, M. (1998) *Low cost but acceptable: A minimum income standard for the UK*, Bristol: The Policy Press and Zacchaeus Trust for the Family Budget Unit.

Pickett, K.E., Kelly, S., Brunner, E., Lobstein, T. and Wilkinson, R.G. (2005) 'Wider income gaps, wider waistbands? An ecological study of obesity and income inequality', *Journal of Epidemiology and Community Health*, vol 59, no 8, pp 670-4.

Pomerleau, J., McKee, M., Lobstein, T. and Knai, C. (2003) 'The burden of disease attributable to nutrition in Europe', *Public Health Nutrition*, vol 6, no 5, pp 453-61.

Prättälä, R., Roos, G., Hulshof, K. and Sihto, M. (2002) 'Food and nutrition policies and interventions', in J. Mackenbach and M. Bakker (eds) *Reducing inequalities in health: A European perspective*, London: Routledge, pp 104-24.

Prentice, A.M. and Jebb, S.A. (2003) 'Fast foods, energy density and obesity: a possible mechanistic link', *Obesity Reviews*, vol 4, no 4, pp 187-94.

Riches, G. (2003) 'Food banks and food security: welfare reform, human rights and social policy. Lessons from Canada?' in E. Dowler and C. Jones Finer (eds) *The welfare of food: Rights and responsibilities in a changing world*, Oxford: Blackwell Publishing, pp 91-105.

Riley, A. (2005) *School meals: Factsheet*, London: Child Poverty Action Group (www.cpag.org.uk, follow links to campaigns).

Robertson, A., Tirado, C., Lobstein, T., Jermini, M., Knai, C., Jensen, J.H., Ferro-Luzzi, A. and James, W.P.T. (eds) (2004) *Food and health in Europe: A new basis for action*, WHO Regional Publications. European Series no 96, Copenhagen: WHO Regional Office for Europe.

Roos, G., Prättälä, R., and FAIR-97-3096 Disparities Group (tasks 4 and 5) (1999) *Disparities in food habits: Review of research in 15 European countries*, Helsinki: National Public Health Institute.

Schäfer Elinder, L., Jossens, L., Raw, M., Andreasson, S. and Lang. T. (2003) *Public health aspects of the EU Common Agricultural Policy: Developments and recommendations for change in four sectors: Fruit and vegetables, dairy, wine and tobacco*, Stockholm: National Institute of Public Health.

Scottish Executive (2005) *The Scottish Health Survey 2003,* Edinburgh: Scottish Executive.

Scottish Office (1994) *The Scottish diet. Report of the Scottish Health Service Advisory Council Working Group on the Scottish Diet chaired by Philip James*, Edinburgh: The Scottish Office.

SEU (Social Exclusion Unit) (2001) *The new commitment to neighbourhood renewal: National Strategy Action Plan*, London: HMSO.

Short, F. (2006) *Kitchen secrets: The meaning of cooking in everyday life*, Oxford: Berg.

Stamatakis, E., Primatesta, P., Chinn, S., Rona, R. and Flascheti, E. (2005) 'Overweight and obesity trends from 1974-2003 in English children: what is the role of socioeconomic factors?', *Archives of Diseases of Childhood*, vol 90, no 10, pp 999-1004.

Sturm, R. and Datar, A. (2005) 'Body Mass Index in elementary school children, metropolitan area food prices and food outlet density', *Public Health*, vol 119, no 12, pp 1059-68.

Sustain and the UK Food Group (2002) *The CAP doesn't fit: Sustain and UK Food Group recommendations for reform of the Common Agricultural Policy*, London: Sustain.

Turrell, G., Hewitt, B., Patterson, C. and Oldenburg, B. (2002) 'Measuring socio-economic position in dietary research: is choice of socio-economic indicator important?' *Public Health Nutrition*, vol 6, no 2, pp 191-200.

Wang, Y. and Lobstein, T. (2006) 'Worldwide trends in childhood overweight and obesity', *International Journal of Pediatric Obesity*, vol 1, no 1, pp 11-25.

Wanless, D. (2002) *Securing our future health: Taking a long-term view. Final report*, London: HM Treasury (www.hm-treasury.gov.uk/consultations_and_legislation/wanless/consult_wanless_final.cfm).

Wanless, D. (2004) *Securing good health for the whole population. Final report*, London: HMSO (www.hm-treasury.gov.uk/consultations_and_legislation/wanless/consult_wanless04_final.cfm).

Wardle, J., Waller, J. and Jarvis, M.J. (2002) 'Sex differences in the association of socioeconomic status with obesity', *Americal Journal of Public Health*, vol 92, no 8, pp 1299-304.

White, M., Bunting, J., Williams, E., Raybould, S., Adamson, A. and Mathers, J.C. (2004) *Do 'food deserts' exist? A multi-level, geographical analysis of the relationship between retail food access, socio-economic position and dietary intake*, London: Food Standards Agency.

WHO and FAO (World Health Organization and Food and Agriculture Organisation) (2003) *Diet, nutrition and the prevention of chronic diseases: Report of a joint WHO/FAO expert consultation*, WHO Technical Report Series No 916, Geneva and Rome: WHO and FAO.

Wrieden, W.L., Anderson, A.S., Longbottom, P.J., Valentine, K., Stead, M., Caraher, M., Lang, T., Gray, B. and Dowler, E. (2007) 'The impact of a community-based food skills intervention on cooking confidence, food preparation methods and dietary choices – an exploratory trial', *Public Health Nutrition*, vol 10, no 2, pp 203-11.

Wrieden, W.L., Barton, K.L., Armstrong, J. and McNeill, G. (2006) *A review of food consumption and nutrient intakes from national surveys in Scotland: Comparison to the Scottish dietary targets*, Aberdeen: Food Standards Agency Scotland.

Wrigley, N. (2002) '"Food deserts" in British cities: policy context and research priorities', *Urban Studies*, vol 39, no 11, pp 2020-4.

Wrigley, N., Warm, D. and Margetts, B. (2003) 'Deprivation, diet, and food retail access: findings from the Leeds "Food Deserts" study', *Environment and Planning A*, vol 35, no 1, pp 151-88.

# NINE

# Behaving badly? Smoking and the role of behaviour change in tackling health inequalities

*Nick Spencer*

## Introduction

Changing health behaviour is a prominent theme in both government health policy and professional practice and, prior to 1997, formed the basis of the government's strategy for addressing health inequalities, or health variations as they were then officially known (Warden, 1995). By 1998, it appeared that the emphasis had shifted from changing behaviour to changing the underlying material and structural conditions associated with both adverse health behaviours and poor health among the disadvantaged. The New Labour government accepted the conclusions of the Acheson Inquiry (Acheson, 1998), echoing those of the Black Report (Townsend and Davidson, 1982), that tackling health inequalities required attention to the structural and material factors underpinning health-related behaviours if they were to be changed. Acheson identified reducing poverty and improving material circumstances as key planks of policy to reducing health inequalities in England. Health behaviour change, including the promotion of smoking cessation, improvement of diet and nutrition and promotion of breastfeeding, was included in the recommendations but set within the social and material context in which health behaviour occurs (see Chapter Eight in this volume for a detailed discussion of dietary and nutritional issues in relation to health inequalities). Government publications explicitly recognised that sustained action on the wider determinants of health would be needed if health inequalities were to be significantly reduced (HM Treasury and DH, 2002). The recent public health White Paper, *Choosing health: Making healthier choices easier* (DH, 2004), however, represents a shift away from materialist explanations of health inequalities by placing health behaviour change at the forefront of public health policy. As the title of the White Paper suggests, its objective is to help the public to 'choose' better health and less emphasis is placed on policy initiatives to address the wider determinants of health inequalities (see Chapters Three, Four, Five and Eight for further discussion of the policy shift represented by *Choosing health*).

Against the background of this shifting policy agenda, this chapter offers an overview of recent health policy initiatives aimed at smoking reduction and the theoretical debates on the effectiveness of policies that seek to reduce health inequalities through changing individual smoking behaviour. Using cigarette smoking as an exemplar, it will examine some of the issues that those concerned with health behaviour change face. Cigarette smoking is the major cause of premature and preventable death in England. Despite numerous campaigns and programmes to promote smoking behaviour change, it remains a health behaviour that is extremely resistant to change. This chapter examines the relationship between cigarette smoking and a range of social and material factors that appear to be key determinants of smoking behaviour. In the light of this discussion, it examines how effective current smoking behaviour change programmes are likely to be and identifies the key challenges for future smoking cessation policy.

## Inequalities in smoking behaviour

Since the 1950s and the accumulation of epidemiological evidence for the health hazards associated with smoking, cigarette smoking has become increasingly socially patterned with high rates of current smoking, heavy consumption and low rates of quitting associated with material and social disadvantage (Townsend et al, 1994; Graham and Der, 1999). Table 9.1 shows the latest data on current smoking by sex and socioeconomic group for Great Britain. Against an overall trend towards reduced cigarette smoking between 2001/02 and 2004/05, the absolute difference in smoking rates between men in higher professional occupations (the group with the lowest rates) and men in routine manual occupations fell from 21% to 17%, while, among women, the absolute difference increased from 20% to 22%.

As footnote 2 in the table indicates, the most disadvantaged social groups are not included. Based on analysis of the General Household Survey and using a cumulative measure of deprivation including occupation, educational level, housing tenure, car ownership, unemployment, overcrowding and single parenthood, Richardson (2001) shows much more striking differences in smoking prevalence between the least and the most deprived groups of the population (see Figure 9.1).

**Table 9.1: Prevalence of cigarette smoking by sex and socioeconomic classification**

| Great Britain | Men (%) | | Women (%) | |
|---|---|---|---|---|
| | 2001/02 | 2004/05 | 2001/02 | 2004/5 |
| *Managerial and professional*[1] | | | | |
| Large employers and higher managerial occupations | 16 | 19 | 15 | 13 |
| Higher professional occupations | 17 | 16 | 13 | 11 |
| Lower managerial and professional occupations | 24 | 22 | 20 | 20 |
| *Intermediate*[1] | | | | |
| Intermediate occupations | 28 | 26 | 26 | 22 |
| Small employers/own account workers | 30 | 25 | 26 | 20 |
| *Routine and manual*[1] | | | | |
| Lower supervisory and technical occupations | 33 | 30 | 29 | 26 |
| Semi-routine occupations | 33 | 34 | 32 | 30 |
| Routine occupations | 38 | 33 | 33 | 33 |
| All people[2] | 28 | 26 | 26 | 23 |

*Notes:*
[1] Classification of the household reference person. See Appendix, Part 1: National Statistics
Socio-economic Classification.
[2] Where the household reference person was a full-time student, had an inadequately described occupation, had never worked or was long-term unemployed these are not shown as separate categories, but are included in the figure for all people aged 16 and over.
*Source:* Babb et al (2006, p 107)

Figure 9.1 further suggests that smoking prevalence among the poorest group of the population changed little between 1973 and 1998. Data from the Scottish Health Survey 2003 show an increase in absolute difference in smoking prevalence when area of deprivation is used compared with occupational group (Scottish Executive, 2005). Nicotine dependency, measured by time to first cigarette during the day and perceived difficulty of going for a whole day without smoking as well as salivary cotinine levels, an objective measure of smoke intake, shows a marked gradient with increasing deprivation score (Richardson, 2001). In studies of smoking households with infants (Blackburn et al, 2003) and toddlers (Spencer et al, 2005), mothers' salivary cotinine levels are socially patterned by income. Daily consumption is closely linked to

**Figure 9.1: Smoking prevalence (both sexes) by cumulative deprivation score, Great Britain, 1973-98**

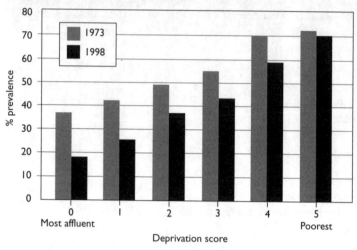

*Source:* Richardson (2001, p 8)

nicotine dependency. A study of nine European countries, including the UK, reported a social gradient in daily consumption by education level (Giskes et al, 2005).

While current socioeconomic status is a powerful, independent indicator of smoking status, life-course socioeconomic position also appears to have an effect independent of current socioeconomic status (Graham and Der, 1999; Gilman et al, 2003; Jefferis et al, 2004). For women, there is an additional independent effect of domestic life course, characterised by age of leaving full-time education and by whether, and at what age, women had become mothers (Graham et al, 2006). Pregnancy, early childhood and adolescence are sensitive periods in the life course. Inequalities by socioeconomic position in smoking in pregnancy contribute to health inequalities in infancy, later childhood and adulthood. Disadvantaged women are much more likely to smoke in pregnancy, are much less likely to quit and are more likely to smoke heavily (Graham, 2003; Spencer, 2003). There is a well-documented social gradient in exposure of infants and young children to cigarette smoke (Blackburn et al, 2003; Spencer et al, 2005) that is likely to have lasting effects. Amongst adolescents, the social gradient is less marked as adolescent smoking is a mark of rebellion (Jarvis, 2004). However, as Jarvis states:

> Children who are attracted to this adolescent assertion of
> perceived adulthood or rebelliousness tend to come from

backgrounds that favour smoking (for example, with high levels of smoking in parents, siblings and peers; relatively deprived neighbourhoods; schools where smoking is common). (Jarvis, 2004, p 277)

This is supported by evidence that young people from social class V are more likely to smoke by age 15 compared with those from social class I (DH, 2004). Heavier smoking is associated with disadvantage in adolescence (Sweeting and West, 2001).

The foregoing discussion concerns only social inequalities. In the UK, there are marked differences in cigarette smoking by ethnic group (see also Chapter Six in this volume for a discussion of the relationship of ethnicity to smoking and other health-related behaviours). Rates in 1999 were high among Bangladeshi men (42%), Irish men (39%), and Black Caribbean men (34%) (Petersen and Peto, 2004). Irish women had rates higher than the general population but Bangladeshi and Black Caribbean women had low rates (Petersen and Peto, 2004). For most of the past 30 years, men have been more likely to smoke than women; however, prevalence rates had almost converged by 2001 and, among young people aged 15-19 years, smoking prevalence was higher among women (31%) compared with men (29%) (Petersen and Peto, 2004).

## Explanations for inequalities in smoking behaviour

Social inequalities in smoking are a relatively recent phenomenon and have emerged particularly in the past 20-30 years (Graham, 1996; Jarvis, 2004). Smokers in higher social groups have tended to quit more readily, whereas quitting appears to be less easy among lower social groups (Jarvis, 2004). Part of the explanation for this may be that nicotine is highly addictive and nicotine intake is strongly correlated with social disadvantage (Jarvis, 2004). This implies that greater will power and support is required for those in disadvantaged circumstances to quit compared with their more privileged peers.

The behaviourist explanation, which was strongly reflected in government publications related to health inequalities or variations prior to 1997 and which has resurfaced in *Choosing health* (DH, 2004), holds that social differences in smoking and other health-related behaviours arise because of ignorance and poorly informed choices. *Choosing health* is explicit in relating health inequalities to 'the cumulative results of thousands of choices by millions of people that impact on health' (DH, 2004, p 15). In this paradigm, socially disadvantaged people are seen as complicit in their own health problems and in need of guidance and education in order to change their behaviour (see Chapters Four and Eight in this volume for further discussion of this paradigm). A sub-set of this explanation is the concept of a 'culture of poverty', in which family health-related behaviours are reinforced and passed from generation to generation. Empirical support for this explanation comes from the finding that children are three times more likely to become smokers themselves if both parents smoke than if neither do (cited in Richardson, 2001).

The materialist/structuralist explanation, broadly endorsed by both the Black and Acheson Reports, holds that the material conditions of people's lives and societal structures influence their behaviours in such a way as to override, limit and mould individual choice (see Chapter Four for further discussion of the materialist explanations of health inequalities). Smoking, although exacting a heavy economic cost on the individual and household, is seen as providing a means of coping with the stresses and strains of living in financially disadvantaged circumstances (Graham, 1993), as well as offering a relatively cheap leisure activity. Smoking among women is also closely linked to caring responsibilities (Graham, 1993).

Recent life-course research adds a further dimension to the materialist/structuralist explanation, showing that social circumstances in early life impact on smoking in early adulthood (Graham and Der, 1999; Gilman et al, 2003; Jefferis et al, 2004). A study based on Finnish longitudinal data illustrates how health-related behaviour is fashioned by early life experience (Lynch et al, 1997). Smoking in pregnancy has also been shown to be influenced by cumulative social exposures in early childhood mediated through socially patterned risk factors around the time of conception (Spencer, 2006).

## Policy interventions to reduce inequalities in smoking behaviour

The Acheson Report made recommendations for policies that promote the adoption of healthier lifestyles, particularly in respect of factors that show a strong social gradient in prevalence or consequences. Specifically, it recommended:

- policies to reduce tobacco smoking, including restricting smoking in public places; abolishing tobacco advertising and promotion; and community, mass media and educational initiatives;
- increases in the real price of tobacco to discourage young people from becoming habitual smokers and to encourage adult smokers to

quit. These increases should be introduced in tandem with policies to improve the living standards of low-income households and policies to help smokers in these households become and remain ex-smokers;

- making nicotine replacement therapy available on prescription.

These specific recommendations were set within a policy context that emphasised the need to reduce the material and structural factors promoting inequalities in health and health-related behaviours such as smoking. Policy responses to the specific recommendations of the Acheson Inquiry are outlined below and discussed in relation to their likely effect on inequalities in health and smoking behaviour.

The Scottish Executive introduced a total ban on smoking in enclosed public spaces in March 2006.[1] The Westminster government, responsible for legislation in England, initially introduced a Bill enacting a partial ban on smoking in public places where food was being served.[2] Following a public debate and severe criticism, including the suggestion that the partial ban would increase inequalities in smoking (Woodall et al, 2005), the Bill has been strengthened and a complete ban on smoking in restaurants and pubs was introduced in July 2007.[3]

The Westminster government's ambivalence on the issue of a total ban on smoking in enclosed public spaces reflected sensitivity about accusations of 'nanny statism' from sections of the press. In addition, New Labour's reluctance to confront powerful interests associated with tobacco advertising was revealed very early by the Bernie Ecclestone scandal[4] in 1997, in which it was alleged that the total ban on tobacco sponsorship of sport was modified to exempt Formula 1 racing under pressure from Ecclestone, who had donated large sums to the Labour Party. However, again under considerable public pressure, the 2002 Tobacco Advertising and Promotion Act[5] banned almost all tobacco advertising except within shops. In 2005, internet advertising and brand sharing (using a non-tobacco product to promote tobacco) were banned.

The government has also made extensive use of media campaigns[6] that have the following aims:

- **motivation:** provides smokers with new and motivating reasons to quit;
- **support:** outlines the choice of NHS support available;
- **reducing exposure to second-hand smoke:** demonstrates that second-hand smoke is dangerous, not just unpleasant;

- **product and pack:** links the health messages back to the product, giving the smoker another reason to quit.

In 2005, the government claimed that advertising was the biggest single prompt to smoking cessation and that the campaign generated nearly 400,000 calls to the NHS Smoking Helpline and nearly 600,000 visits to the campaign website (www.givingupsmoking.co.uk).

In addition to media campaigns and the helpline, the government set up in 2003 the NHS Stop Smoking Service and a nicotine replacement therapy (NRT) service.[7] Counselling and support services complement the use of NRT and the drug bupropion that are available on prescription.

A behaviour change model, known as the transtheoretical (stages of change) model (TTM), has been promoted as an effective method of smoking cessation in populations (Prochaska and Velicer, 2004). TTM is based on a theory of behaviour change in which individuals are classified according to their stage of readiness to change. The model has been used extensively in clinical trials in the US and elsewhere and has been incorporated into training materials for health professionals in the UK (HEA, 1997).

In July 1997, New Labour announced its intention to raise tobacco taxes by 5% above inflation every year.[8] The commitment was carried out in 1998 and 1999 but abandoned in 2000. In subsequent years, tobacco taxes have risen in line with inflation. Increases in tobacco prices disproportionately affect those on low incomes as the less well off spend more of their income on cigarettes than those on high incomes. In fact, it has been argued that increasing tobacco prices exacerbates health inequalities rather than reducing them as it has least effect among those on low income (Marsh and Mackay, 1994).

Although steps have been taken in relation to tobacco that are in line with the recommendations of the Acheson Inquiry, the *Choosing health* White Paper (DH, 2004) represents a significant move back towards a behaviourist approach to health inequalities and away from the materialist/structuralist paradigm favoured by Acheson. While paying lip service to the need to eradicate poverty and disadvantage, the overwhelming message of the White Paper is that health is a matter of individual choice and health inequalities arise because those who are more disadvantaged make more unhealthy choices. The White Paper acknowledges that government has a role in enabling healthier choices to be made but the responsibility for public health is seen as resting firmly with individuals. Consistent with this view is the proposal to appoint 'health trainers', particularly in disadvantaged areas, to advise people on healthy lifestyles (see also Chapters Three and Four of this volume). 'Health trainers' will be drawn from local communities and will be accredited by the NHS. They will provide support for people to make informed lifestyle choices.

Policies aimed at reducing social exclusion and increasing the income of the disadvantaged are likely to have an impact on inequalities in health behaviour. Economic growth, combined with fiscal policies such as the minimum wage, has led to improvements in employment and in the material circumstances of many households (Hills and Stewart, 2005).

## Evidence for effectiveness of policies and interventions in reducing inequalities in smoking

There is reasonable evidence of the effectiveness of bans on smoking in public places. A systematic Cochrane review (Serra et al, 2000) found 11 studies, all uncontrolled before and after studies, and they conclude that these interventions result in reduction in smoking in public places. Community interventions to reduce smoking among adults have not been shown to be effective (Secker-Walker et al, 2002) but there is some limited evidence that community-level interventions can discourage uptake of cigarette smoking among young people under 25 years of age (Sowden and Stead, 2003). There is only weak evidence that mass media campaigns deter uptake of cigarette smoking among young people (Sowden and Arblaster, 1998).

At the individual level, nicotine replacement therapy has been shown to be effective in helping smokers to quit (Silagy et al, 2004). Both telephone (Stead et al, 2006) and physician (Lancaster and Stead, 2004) counselling have been shown to positively contribute to smoking cessation. The evidence for stage of change approaches to smoking cessation has not been systematically reviewed. The creators of the transtheoretical (stages of change) model argue that it is more effective than standard methods of behaviour change because it allows practitioners to target those who are ready to change (Prochaska and Velicer, 2004). A cluster randomised trial in the UK comparing the effectiveness of stage of change interventions with standard care in smoking cessation in pregnancy reported a small borderline increase in quitting in the stage of change intervention groups compared with the standard care controls. However, the authors conclude that 'given that the intervention was resource intensive, it is of doubtful benefit' (Lawrence et al, 2003, p 176). In addition to having only a marginal benefit over standard care, the stages of change model, when applied in early pregnancy, has been shown in the UK context to be strongly influenced by social factors. Women in early pregnancy were shown to be much more likely to be in the first, pre-contemplation, stage if they were on income support (Batten et al, 1999). This would suggest that if this model were applied across populations as suggested by Prochaska and Velicer (2004), inequalities in smoking would be likely to increase rather than decrease.

Despite the evidence for effectiveness of policies and interventions aimed at preventing smoking or assisting cessation, there is very little evidence that these policies and interventions reduce inequalities in smoking. A review of systematic reviews and meta-analyses undertaken by the Health Development Agency (HDA, 2004) found no review-level evidence of effective interventions to reduce inequalities, although studies have been undertaken into smoking cessation in low-income and disadvantaged groups, particularly in the US.

New Labour policy has included many of the interventions considered earlier, but they are set within the overall philosophy of the public health White Paper (DH, 2004). As discussed earlier and in other chapters in this book (Chapters Three, Four, Five and Eight), the philosophy represents a return to a behaviourist approach to health in general and health inequalities in particular. Smoking, along with other health-related behaviours, is viewed within this paradigm as, primarily, a matter of choice. There are sound theoretical grounds for questioning the effectiveness of this paradigm in reducing health inequalities. First, the behaviourist paradigm runs counter to the vast body of empirical evidence reviewed by the Black and Acheson Reports that health inequalities are not simply the result of the unhealthy lifestyles of poorer people but are embedded within the unequal structure of societies (see also Chapters Four and Eight for further discussion of the structural influences on health and lifestyle). Second, unhealthy lifestyles are not the only or, necessarily, the main determinants of health inequalities. There is well-documented evidence from many studies, notably the Whitehall studies (Marmot et al, 1991), that smoking and other adverse lifestyle factors explain only a limited part of the differences in health outcomes across the social groups. Third, differences in health-related behaviour do not simply arise as a result of ignorance of the health effects of these behaviours. There is a vast body of work showing that knowledge and behaviour do not have a direct relationship and it cannot be assumed that increased knowledge directly translates into changed behaviour. Further, there is little evidence of difference in knowledge about the adverse effects of health-related behaviours between advantaged and disadvantaged groups. As Graham (1993) states in her study of smoking among disadvantaged women:

> ... there seems to be no straightforward connection between knowledge and behaviour: women know about the health risks of smoking in pregnancy but continue to smoke despite that knowledge. The crucial connections lay, instead, in women's material and financial circumstances. (p 101)

There are also grounds for anticipating that the particular form of behaviourist approach adopted by the White Paper, the so-called choice agenda, is more likely to widen rather than reduce inequalities in health and health behaviour. The choice agenda presupposes that everyone has an equal opportunity to choose and that health is anyway a matter of choice. The reality, documented in numerous publications, is quite different; health and behaviours associated with health are embedded in social circumstances and social circumstances become 'embodied' in the biology of individuals who experience them (Krieger, 2005). People do not choose the early life experiences that play an important role in forming their life trajectories and their future patterns of health and disease.

Choice, in so far as it exists in relation to health, is hedged around by a multitude of financial, social, environmental, and cultural constraints. For example, Richardson (2001), when discussing strategies for reducing inequalities in smoking, cites a qualitative Scottish study (Stead et al, 1999) that concluded:

> A poorly resourced and stressful environment, strong community norms, isolation from wider societal norms, and limited opportunities for respite and recreation appear to combine not only to foster smoking but also to discourage or undermine cessation. (Cited in Richardson, 2001, p 15)

## Challenges for future smoking cessation policy

Smoking has been a major focus of public health policy for more than 20 years. New Labour has continued that focus and has strengthened some evidence-based interventions, such as nicotine replacement therapy, that have been shown to be effective in smoking cessation. Many of these initiatives have been directed at disadvantaged areas, although clear evidence for their success in reducing inequalities in smoking prevalence rates is lacking. The weak evidence base for interventions aimed at reducing inequalities in lifestyle factors that are detrimental to health means that, as Asthana and Halliday (2006) point out:

> ... there is a lack of understanding of the very features that might make such intervention appropriate for vulnerable groups and those with multiple risks – what would increase smoking cessation among heavy smokers and women of lower socio-economic class, for example? (p 462)

The continued provision and extension of these interventions is likely to result in a decline in smoking prevalence generally; however, new approaches will be needed if the current inequalities in smoking rates are to be reduced. The main challenge lies in the philosophy underpinning public health strategies. As discussed above, the choice agenda outlined in *Choosing health* (DH, 2004) is likely to exacerbate rather than reduce health inequalities. In the presence of increasing inequalities in income distribution (see Chapter Four for a fuller discussion of the role of income inequalities), strategies based on individual choice are unlikely to overcome the structural forces promoting inequalities in health and health-related behaviour.

Policies directly addressing these structural and material forces are likely to be necessary if inequalities are to be reduced. As Graham et al (2006) conclude:

> ... public health policies should be widened beyond their traditional focus on changing individual behaviour, to moderating the unequal lifecourse pathways in which smoking careers are embedded. This broader vision of tobacco control policy would include evaluation of policies that influence children's exposure to disadvantage, the life chances of young people heading for early school leaving and early parenthood, and the social and material circumstances of women, particularly lone mothers, whose employment opportunities are restricted to the low waged sectors of the labour market. (p 232)

Alternative strategies will need to:

- revisit the theoretical and philosophical basis of public health policy and reassert the key role of structural and material factors as determinants of health and health-related behaviour;

- include policies to reduce income inequalities and ensure that all citizens, whether employed or not, have incomes sufficient to allow them access to the goods and services taken for granted by the majority of the population;
- strengthen current initiatives such as the NHS Stop Smoking Service and NRT and ensure that sufficient resources are available in areas of deprivation to address the specific problems of poor uptake of services among these groups. This might need to include innovative approaches such as outreach services to pubs, clubs and homes in disadvantaged areas;
- commission a programme of research to provide evidence of effective interventions in relation to smoking cessation and harm reduction among disadvantaged groups. Such an approach would need to use the framework for trials of complex interventions developed by the Medical Research Council (MRC, 2000) that identifies five phases of study: a theory phase to explore relevant theory; a modelling phase to identify the components of the intervention; an exploratory trial phase to develop a feasible protocol and describe the components of a replicable intervention; a definitive trial phase comparing a fully defined intervention with an appropriate alternative; and a long-term implementation phase to determine if the intervention can be replicated over the long term.

## Conclusion

This chapter has addressed inequalities in health-related behaviour using smoking as an exemplar. The conclusions that can be drawn from the above discussion apply equally to inequalities in other aspects of health-related behaviour such as nutrition and exercise. The essential message is that such behaviours are not simply the result of choice but are embedded in the social circumstances of people's lives and are influenced by their life-course circumstances and experiences. Reducing these inequalities will require much more than interventions aimed at helping people to make the right choices. Policy measures to reduce the adverse social circumstances in which these behaviours flourish are needed alongside the range of interventions that government is already making to inform and assist behaviour change.

## Notes

[1,2] www.news.bbc.co.uk/1/hi/health/4014597.stm (accessed 26 August 2006).

[3] www.thesite.org/drinkanddrugs/drugsafety/smoking/smokingban (accessed 26 August 2006).

[4] www.news.bbc.co.uk/1/hi/uk_politics/937232.stm (accessed 26 August 2006).

[5] www.opsi.gov.uk/acts/en2002/2002en36.htm (accessed 26 August 2006).

[6] www.dh.gov.uk/PolicyandGuidance/HealthandSocialCaretopics/ Tobacco/TobaccoGeneralInformation/TobaccoGeneralArticle/fs/ en?CONTENT_ID=1426098&chk=rZybbX (accessed 26 August 2006).

[7] www.dh.gov.uk/PolicyandGuidance/HealthandSocialCaretopics/ Tobacco/TobaccoGeneralInformation/TobaccoGeneralArticle/fs/ en?CONTENT_ID=4002192&chk=5Xx9q6 (accessed 26 August 2006).

[8] www.ash.org.uk/html/factsheets/html/fact16.html (accessed 26 August 2006).

## References

Acheson, D. (1998) *Independent inquiry into inequalities in health*, London: The Stationery Office.

Asthana, S. and Halliday, J. (2006) *What works in tackling health inequalities: Pathways, policies and practice across the lifecourse*, Bristol: The Policy Press.

Babb, P., Butcher, H., Church, J. and Zealey, L. (eds) (2006) *Social Trends No 36 – 2006 edition*, London: Palgrave Macmillan for Office of National Statistics.

Batten, L., Graham, H., High, S., Ruggiero, L. and Rossi, J. (1999) 'State of change, low income and benefit status: a profile of women's smoking in early pregnancy', *Health Education Journal*, vol 58, no 4, pp 378-88.

Blackburn, C., Spencer, N., Bonas, S., Coe, C., Dolan, A. and Moy, R. (2003) 'Effect of strategies to reduce exposure of infants to environmental tobacco smoke in the home: cross sectional survey', *BMJ*, vol 327, pp 257-9.

DH (Department of Health) (2004) *Choosing health: Making healthier choices easier*, Cm 6374, London: The Stationery Office.

Gilman, S.E., Abrams, D.B. and Buka, S.L. (2003) 'Socioeconomic status over the life course and stages of cigarette use: initiation, regular use, and cessation', *Journal of Epidemiology and Community Health*, vol 57, no 10, pp 802-8.

Giskes, K., Kunst, A.E., Benach, J., Borrell, C., Costa, G., Dahl, E., Dalstra, J.A., Federico, B., Helmert, U., Judge, K., Lahelma, E., Moussa, K., Ostergren, P.O., Platt, S., Prattala, R., Rasmussen, N.K. and Mackenbach, J.P. (2005) 'Trends in smoking behaviour between 1985 and 2000 in nine European countries by education', *Journal of Epidemiology and Community Health*, vol 59, no 5, pp 395-401.

Graham, H. (1993) *When life's a drag: Women, smoking and disadvantage*, London: HMSO.

Graham, H. (1996) 'Smoking prevalence among women in the European Community, 1950-1990', *Social Science and Medicine*, vol 43, no 2, pp 243-54.

Graham, H. (2003) 'Disadvantaged lives and women's smoking: patterns and policy levers', *MIDIRS Midwifery Digest*, vol 13, no 2, pp 152-6.

Graham, H., and Der, G. (1999) 'Patterns and predictors of tobacco consumption among women', *Health Education Research*, vol 14, no 5, pp 611-18.

Graham, H., Francis, B., Inskip, H.M., Harman, J. and the Southampton Women's Study Group (2006) 'Socioeconomic lifecourse influences on women's smoking status in early adulthood', *Journal of Epidemiology and Community Health*, vol 60, no 3, pp 228-33.

HDA (Health Development Agency) (2004) *Smoking and public health: A review of reviews of interventions to increase smoking cessation, reduce smoking initiation, and prevent further uptake of smoking*, London: HDA.

HEA (Health Education Authority) (1997) *Helping people change trainers' manual*, London: HEA.

Hills, J. and Stewart, K. (eds) (2005) *A more equal society? New Labour, poverty, inequality and exclusion*, Bristol: The Policy Press.

HM Treasury and DH (2002) *Tackling health inequalities: Summary of the 2002 cross-cutting review*, London: DH.

Jarvis, M.J. (2004) 'Why people smoke', *BMJ*, vol 328, pp 277-9.

Jefferis, B., Power, C. and Graham, H. (2004) 'Effects of childhood socioeconomic circumstances on persistent smoking', *American Journal of Public Health*, vol 94, no 2, pp 279-85.

Krieger, N. (2005) 'Embodiment: a conceptual glossary for epidemiology', *Journal of Epidemiology and Community Health*, vol 59, no 5, pp 350-5.

Lancaster, T. and Stead, L.F. (2004) 'Physician advice for smoking cessation', *Cochrane Database of Systematic Reviews*, Issue 4, Art No CD000165. DOI:10.1002/14651858. CD000165.

Lawrence, T., Aveyard, P., Evans, O. and Cheng, K.K. (2003) 'A cluster randomised controlled trial of smoking cessation in pregnant women comparing interventions based on the transtheoretical (stages of change) model to standard care', *Tobacco Control*, vol 12, no 2, pp 168-77.

Lynch, J.W., Kaplan, G.A. and Salonen, J.T. (1997) 'Why do poor people behave poorly? Variation in adult health behaviours and psychosocial characteristics by stages of the socioeconomic lifecourse', *Social Science and Medicine*, vol 44, no 6, pp 809-19.

Marmot, M.G., Smith, G.D., Stansfeld, S., Patel, C., North, F., Head, J., White, I., Brunner, E. and Feeney, A. (1991) 'Health inequalities among British civil servants: the Whitehall II study', *Lancet*, vol 337, no S754, pp 1387-93.

Marsh, A. and McKay, S. (1994) *Poor smokers*, London: Policy Studies Institute.

MRC (Medical Research Council) (2000) *A framework for development and evaluation of RCTs for complex interventions to improve health*, London: MRC.

Petersen, S. and Peto, V. (2004) *Smoking statistics 2004*, London: British Heart Foundation.

Prochaska, J.O. and Velicer, W.F. (2004) 'Integrating population smoking cessation policies and programs', *Public Health Reports*, vol 119, no 3, pp 244-52.

Richardson, K. (2001) *Smoking, low income and health inequalities: Thematic discussion document*, London: Action for Smoking and Health and Health Development Agency.

Scottish Executive (2005) *Scottish Health Survey 2003: Summary of key findings*, Edinburgh: Scottish Executive.

Secker-Walker, R.H., Gnich, W., Platt, S. and Lancaster, T. (2002) 'Community interventions for reducing smoking among adults', *Cochrane Database of Systematic Reviews*, Issue 2, Art No CD001745. DOI:10.1002/14651858. CD001745.

Serra, C., Cabezas, C., Bonfill, X. and Padeval-Vila, M. (2000) 'Interventions for preventing smoking in public places', *Cochrane Database of Systematic Reviews*, Issue 3, Art No CD001294. DOI:10.1002/14651858. CD001294.

Silagy, C., Lancaster, T., Stead, L., Mant, D. and Fowler, G. (2004) 'Nicotine replacement therapy for smoking cessation', *Cochrane Database of Systematic Reviews*, Issue 3, Art No CD000146. DOI:10.1002/14651858. CD000146, pub2.

Sowden, A.J. and Arblaster, L. (1998) 'Mass media interventions for preventing smoking in young people', *Cochrane Database of Systematic Reviews*, Issue 4, Art No CD001006. DOI:10.1002/14651858. CD001006.

Sowden, A. and Stead, L. (2003) 'Community interventions for preventing smoking in young people', *Cochrane Database of Systematic Reviews,* Issue 1, Art No CD001291. DOI:10.1002/14651858. CD001291.

Spencer, N.J. (2003) *Weighing the evidence: How birthweight is determined*, Abingdon: Radcliffe Press.

Spencer, N.J. (2006) 'Explaining the social gradient in smoking in pregnancy: early life course accumulation and cross-sectional clustering of social risk exposures in the 1958 British national cohort', *Social Science and Medicine*, vol 62, no 5, pp 1250-9.

Spencer, N.J., Blackburn, C., Bonas, S., Dolan, A., and Coe, C.J. (2005) 'Home smoking ban and toddler (18-30 months) smoke exposure: a cross sectional study', *Archives of Disease in Childhood*, vol 90, pp 670-4.

Stead, L.F., Perera, R. and Lancaster, T. (2006) 'Telephone counselling for smoking cessation' *Cochrane Database of Systematic Reviews*, Issue 3, Art No CD002850. DOI:10.1002/14651858. CD002850.pub2.

Stead, M., MacAskill, S., MacKintosh, A.-M., Reece, J. and Eadie, D. (1999) *An investigation into smoking cessation in disadvantaged communities: Qualitative focus group research*, Glasgow: Centre for Tobacco Control Research, University of Strathclyde.

Sweeting, H. and West, P. (2001) 'Social class and smoking at age 15: the effect of different definitions of smoking', *Addiction*, vol 96, no 9, pp 1357-9.

Townsend, P. and Davidson, N. (1982) *Inequalities in health: The Black Report*, Harmondsworth:Penguin.

Townsend, J., Roderick, P. and Cooper, J. (1994) 'Cigarette smoking by socio-economic group, sex, and age: effects of price, income and health publicity', *BMJ*, vol 309, pp 923-7.

Warden, J. (1995) 'UK government will fund research into health variations', *BMJ*, vol 311, p 1119.

Woodall, A.A., Sandbach, E.J., Woodward, C.M., Aveyard, P. and Merrington, G. (2005) 'The partial smoking ban in licensed establishments and health inequalities in England: modelling study', *BMJ*, vol 331, pp 488-9.

# TEN

# Health inequalities and user involvement

*Jonathan Tritter and Helen Lester*

## Introduction

Patient and public involvement has been suggested as a mechanism to engage individuals more fully in their own healthcare and to reorient service provision around the needs of users rather than providers (Tritter and Macallum, 2006). Yet, patterns of health inequality are also reflected in those who tend to be involved and those who are members of 'hard to reach' groups. The Acheson Report (Acheson, 1998) includes no explicit mention of involvement but has had a significant influence in integrating a sensitivity to diversity in most activities seeking to engage patients, carers and members of the public. Unless user involvement draws on the diverse range of the population and aims to be inclusive, it can only serve to reinforce existing patterns of inequality in health provision, access and outcomes.

A key weakness in user involvement[1] is its capacity to result in a 'tyranny of the majority' (Madison, 1961[1787]). Indeed, there is evidence that particular populations are underrepresented in user involvement activities (Clark et al, 2004). The users who participate may be disproportionately those who have experience of services and are best able to engage and present their issues. Therefore greater emphasis on involving users may exacerbate underlying inequalities of access, resources and ability.

This chapter begins by summarising the recent UK policy context and differentiating between types of involvement. It then highlights the problems in trying to define 'hard to reach' groups and the importance of user involvement for such groups. There is a particular focus on the health inequalities experienced by two 'hard to reach' groups – people with serious mental illness and those who are homeless – and examples of successful involvement strategies. The chapter concludes by suggesting that user involvement is everyone's business but requires radical shifts in both theory and practice to succeed.

## The policy context of user involvement

The past 20 years have been characterised by a rapid growth in a range of different user involvement activities underpinned by a multitude of policy directives across all countries of the Organisation for Economic Cooperation and Development. Since the establishment of Community Health Councils in 1973, the rhetoric of user involvement has become a central component of health and social policy in the UK. The 1990 NHS and Community Care Act was the first piece of UK legislation to establish a formal requirement for user involvement in service planning. Subsequent key policies in the early 1990s included *The patient's charter* (DH, 1991) and *Local voices* (NHS Management Executive, 1992), aimed to make services more responsive to patients' needs as consumers. Under New Labour, the user involvement agenda has continued to be formalised in policy terms through *The NHS Plan* (DH, 2000), which emphasised the government's commitment to creating a patient-centred NHS with users' needs central to service design and delivery: 'NHS care has to be shaped around the convenience and concerns of patients. To bring this about, patients must have more say in their own treatment and more influence over the way the NHS works' (DH, 2000, p 88).

New statutory duties placed on NHS organisations by the 2001 Health and Social Care Act now ensure that patients and the public are consulted at an early stage about the planning and organisation of services (DH, 2003b). Patient Advisory and Liaison Services and Patient and Public Involvement Forums have been set up in every NHS trust to provide information and on-site help for patients. A new national network of Independent Complaints Advocacy Services, provided locally but operating to national standards, has been set up to support people when they want to complain about the NHS. More recently, *Creating a patient-led NHS: Delivering the NHS improvement plan* (DH, 2005, p 11) suggested that 'patient and public involvement should be part of everyday practice in the NHS and must lead to action' and that 'some groups of people, including some from black and minority ethnic backgrounds, are difficult to reach, less well-served and less satisfied with services. The NHS needs to make sure it is sensitive to the needs of all groups' (DH, 2005, p 9). The publication of *A stronger local voice* (DH, 2006a) in July 2006 and the government's response in December (DH, 2006b), together with the presentation to Parliament of the Local Government and Patient and Public Involvement in Health Bill, raise the prospect of another structural change to replace Patient and Public Involvement Forums with Local Involvement Networks in each local authority that commissions social services. These new organisations will work across health and social care, play a key role in feeding into inspection and regulation as well as commissioning and be supported by the recently established NHS Centre for Involvement.

The emphasis on user involvement has been driven by a number of different agendas:

- creating accountability to tax-paying citizens;
- consumerist principles and the patient choice agenda;
- a mechanism to increase local accountability within the NHS;
- the promotion of a broader partnership agenda.

Justifications for user involvement in health occupy a continuum between democratic and consumerist models (Croft and Beresford, 1993, 1995; Feldberg and Vipond, 1999). Typically, the distinctions relate to rights inherent in citizenship versus those of individual choice in the marketplace. Since 1948, the NHS has been funded through central taxation and so taxpaying citizens should have a say in what services are funded and how they are delivered. Governments remain concerned with 'value for money' justifications for public spending and increasingly feel the need to strengthen the opportunities for accountability to the voice of the public in decisions about the organisation and delivery of health services.

Healthcare users are often presented as consumers enabled to exercise choice to ensure that their needs are met. More recently, the patient choice agenda, fuelled by the promotion of health markets in the NHS, wider availability of information and a slowly growing private sector (Appleby et al, 2003), has become a particularly strong political imperative. It has generated heated debate, a 'patient tsar' and the government's published response to consultation, *Building on the best* (DH, 2003a), which presents a series of measures to extend patient choice across primary, secondary and community care. User involvement is presented as the most important feedback mechanism for the expression of consumer views, an essential component of markets. However, to be consumers, patients must have the necessary information to choose, and their choices must change service provision.

The desire to increase the accountability of the NHS and the professionals who work within it is a further strong driver for increased user involvement. Medical practitioners who fail in their duty of care to patients are perhaps best represented in the collective public consciousness by Harold Shipman, the general practitioner found guilty of murdering 15 of his female patients in 2000, and by the unnecessary deaths of up to 35 children under the care of the Bristol

Royal Infirmary paediatric cardiac surgeons. While it is tempting to argue that Shipman has little to do with the reality of healthcare in the UK, the 198 recommendations in the Bristol Royal Infirmary Inquiry (DH, 2001) and other cases have come to symbolise the unchecked autonomy of the medical profession. Allied to a growing momentum within the medical profession to increase accountability, patient and public involvement is now seen as one aspect of the broader clinical governance agenda.

The concept of 'partnership' is a further significant policy driver that is embedded in a range of New Labour policy areas including local government, healthcare, education and crime and disorder. Examples of New Labour's commitment to 'joined-up solutions to joined-up problems' include the duty of partnership between health and social care, joint planning frameworks, new intermediate care services to prevent unnecessary hospital admissions and Health Action Zones to improve the health of local communities in areas of high social exclusion (Poxton, 2003).

## Types of user involvement

Just as the drivers promoting user involvement are varied, there are different categories of user involvement. Patient participation in treatment decisions is one type of user involvement, but, as a form of patient-centred care, is not innovative. Similarly, involvement in service development, typically a consultation exercise with the local community, has a long history in the NHS. The evaluation of services by users has become common practice; simple satisfaction questionnaires, and more robust investigations, are now part of many audit exercises. One final category of user involvement relates to participation in research and teaching.

Clearly, there are interactions and linkages between the different categories of user involvement: service development may have a direct impact on the range of individual treatment options that exist and service evaluation may identify inequities in access that affect individual participation in treatment. User participation in setting a research agenda may have an impact on shaping provision and service organisation, and therefore options for treatment (Involve, 2003).

## Defining 'hard to reach' groups

Reducing inequalities in health and health provision and reaching 'hard to reach' groups is a key theme underpinning many of the more recent NHS White Papers and National Service Frameworks (DH, 2002a). Although health inequalities can affect all communities, they are more likely to be experienced by 'hard to reach' groups that have both poorer access to care and poorer health outcomes. It is difficult, however, to adequately define what is meant by the term 'hard to reach'. Indeed, we suggest that this complex and under-analysed concept has been used inconsistently, and is misleading and potentially stigmatising. The phrase is often used interchangeably with 'underclass', the socially excluded, disengaged, vulnerable, high risk and marginalised. Underpinning each of these terms is a notion of 'otherness' and of groups that are, in some way, problematic for wider society.

The pejorative nature of the term may stem from its use in the 1980s in the context of human immunodeficiency virus (HIV) and acquired immune deficiency syndrome (AIDS). The behaviour of gay men, sex workers and injecting drug users, the groups perceived initially as most at risk of contracting and spreading HIV, was seen as outside the moral boundaries of normal society. The public health agenda focused on trying to 'reach' those who were defined as a threat to the public (and moral) health of the nation and, in doing so, encouraging behaviour modification. Some of the stigmatisation of these groups and the implicit message that they somehow represented 'the out of reach' seemed to reinforce their position on the 'outside'. As Faugier and Sargeant (1997, p 797) suggest, 'social barriers created by ignorance combined with prejudice and discrimination have meant that many of these populations remain marginalized and have restricted access to appropriate health care'.

More recently, the typology of 'hard to reach' groups' used in the 2004 Home Office report *Delivering services to 'hard to reach' families in On Track areas: Definition, consultation and needs assessment* (Doherty, 2004) focuses on three key groups: minority groups (the traditionally underrepresented groups, and the marginalised, disadvantaged or socially excluded, such as travellers or asylum seekers); those 'slipping through the net' (the overlooked, invisible, or those unable to articulate their needs, such as people with mental health problems); and the 'service resistant' who are unwilling to engage with service providers (the suspicious, the over-targeted or disaffected, typically positions attributed to drug users and rough sleepers).

It is also interesting to note that in terms of inaccuracy, 'hard to reach' has sometimes been used to refer to groups that are already engaged but hold challenging views. In the context of improving police relations with 'hard to reach' groups, Jones and Newburn (2001, p 8) argue: 'I'm not sure that these groups are "hard to reach"; some groups are very vociferous, articulate and organised. It's the case of us not liking what we hear, or perhaps just not asking them'. They go on to suggest that the defining characteristics of 'hard to reach' groups include their numerical size and concentration (with smaller and widely dispersed groups harder to access), suspicion of authority, poverty, social invisibility, language barriers, cultural and ideological barriers, and groups with distinctive service needs, such as homeless people. They also warn against a homogenised approach to access and involvement in view of the intrinsic heterogeneity of 'hard to reach' groups.

## Why is user involvement important?

There are a number of, often interrelated, reasons for believing that user involvement is more than a politically mandated 'good thing', related to patients as consumers exerting choice and as taxpayers looking for value for money. User involvement can also be seen as an element of a broader clinical governance agenda, a worthwhile activity with the following practical and ethical benefits:

- users are experts in their own illness and care needs;
- users may have different but equally important perspectives about their illness and care;
- users are able to develop alternative approaches to their illness;
- user involvement may of itself be therapeutic.

Encouraging greater user involvement, including paid activity, can be empowering and address issues of poverty, and therefore may act as one mechanism to encourage greater social inclusion and address some aspects of health inequalities (Sayce and Morris, 1999). Above all, in the context of 'hard to reach' groups, Wilkinson's (1996) arguments, that relative rather than absolute poverty within societies creates health inequalities through mediating factors such as powerlessness and social stress, are critical (see Chapter Four of this volume for a detailed discussion of Wilkinson's arguments).

## Methodologies for engaging 'hard to reach' groups

Policy makers in the UK appear to be more comfortable using predominantly 'top-down' approaches to user involvement. Indeed, the largest consultation exercise on health priorities in the UK to date involved the distribution of 12 million leaflets asking: 'What are the top three things you think would make the NHS better for you and your family?' A *British Medical Journal* editorial commented: 'We need a culture of involvement, not policy making by 12 million leaflets' (Anderson and Florin, 2000, p 1553).

There are a small number of projects that aim to involve the 'hard to reach' and highlight key elements for successful involvement. Common themes appear to be: the importance of taking a 'bottom-up' approach and working at a local level; innovative and multiple ways of working, for example recognising that not everyone is comfortable in group situations; and an understanding that it takes time and effort and perhaps a shift in culture within an organisation to acknowledge the value of user involvement (see Chapter Eleven for a discussion of some of the limitations of local initiatives). Recruiting local users to paid posts, and acknowledging that time spent in activities requires financial recognition, also appear to underpin successful involvement (Edmans and Taket, 2001; Doherty et al, 2004). 'Drop-ins' and informal events in community-based settings are also more likely to reach 'hard to reach' groups than more formal mechanisms of involvement (Cook, 2002). Networking with others who provide services to marginalised groups, drawing on reserves of community knowledge, is also important. Finally, involvement throughout all stages of a consultation process and an ongoing commitment to the group, rather than a 'rubber-stamping' approach to engagement, facilitates successful involvement (HSE, 2004).

## Case study 1: user involvement for people with serious mental illness

People with serious mental illness could be categorised as 'hard to reach' using any of the definitions discussed earlier in this chapter. They are among the most excluded in British society (Sayce, 2001; ODPM, 2004). They have fewer social networks than average, with many of their contacts related to health services rather than sports, family, faith, employment, education or arts and culture. Indeed, one survey found that 40% of people with ongoing mental health problems had no social contacts outside mental health services (Ford et al, 1998).

Perhaps the biggest issue for people with mental health problems is that of unemployment and the consequent risk of financial hardship. In the general working-age population, 70-90% of people are economically active. However, in England, only 24% of people with mental health problems are currently in work, the lowest employment rate of any group of people (ONS, 2002).

People with serious mental illness are also often stereotyped as irrational and violent, creating further barriers in terms of inclusion within wider society (Lester et al, 2005). The reality is that about 95% of violent crime in the UK is committed by people without mental health problems (Sayce, 2000). Indeed, people with mental health problems are more likely to be the victims rather than the perpetrators of crime (Jewesbury, 1998; Sayce, 1997, 1999; McCabe and Ford, 2001; ODPM, 2004). Jonathan Freedland, writing in *The Guardian* in 1998, succinctly captured the consequences of living with mental illness in this country:

> One group in the country has fewer rights than the rest of us. No one listens to what they say, they are mocked in harsh, ugly language and some can't even vote. They can be discriminated at work and locked up even when they have committed no crime. Comedians joke about them, headline writers demonise them and now the Government is set to erode their liberty yet further. They are the mentally ill. (Freedland, 1998, p 17)

In terms of their health, people with serious mental illness have a higher risk of medical illness than the general population and have an increased (two- to fourfold) relative risk of premature death, dying at least 10 years earlier than age-matched contemporaries (Marder et al, 2004; Connolly and Kelly, 2005). The Office for National Statistics survey of psychiatric morbidity among adults living in private households (Singleton et al, 2001) found that 62% of people with psychosis reported a physical condition, compared with 42% of those without psychosis. Diabetes, for example, is up to five times as frequent in patients with schizophrenia and bipolar affective disorder than in the general population (Mukherjee et al, 1996).

Against this background, user involvement in mental health has been encouraged for over a decade (DH, 1992, 1994, 1995) and continues to be an important theme in mental health policy (DH, 2002b). There remains, however something of a rhetoric/reality gap. Wallcraft and Bryant's (2003, p 1) survey of the mental health service user movement in England identified 318 user groups and found that 'local service user groups play a very important role in mutual support, combating stigma, helping people to recover and stay out of services and participating in local service planning and development'. However, most groups were small, recently formed, poorly funded and non-representative of Black and minority ethnic communities, all of which limited their capacity to achieve change. So, while it is true that there are many more user groups than there used to be, it appears that their influence is limited.

### Examples of positive practice in encouraging user involvement for people with serious mental illness

Perhaps the most challenging example of user involvement for people with serious mental illness relates to employing them as part of the paid mental health workforce. There are a small number of locality-based initiatives, such as the St George's Mental Health Trust, which aims to fill at least one quarter of its posts with people with lived experience of mental health services (Perkins et al, 1999). This award-winning service has also, interestingly, led to a net reduction in overall service costs because of savings in state benefit payments and reduced treatment costs. On a national stage, recent mental health workforce developments include the use of support time and recovery (STR) workers (DH, 2003c). STR workers include volunteers and existing and former service users who have the ability to listen to people without judging them. They work as part of a team that provides mental health services, and focus directly on the needs of service users, working across boundaries, providing support, giving time and promoting their recovery.

There is evidence to suggest that involving service users as paid workers is seen as a very positive move by many people who themselves have serious mental illness, and can help them both express their problems and navigate their way through the healthcare system.

> "The things, the experiences, the emotions, the feelings that we as people suffering from mental distress go through simply aren't experienced by people in good health. Trying to get that across to someone who hasn't ever felt like the Sword of Damocles is hanging round your neck for no apparently good reason, you know, you can't do it. It's like trying to explain colours to a blind man. You are trying to explain an emotive language, a set of emotions, which you know you shouldn't have and normal people don't have,

and trying to get these across is an almost impossible task ... I would have found it very useful to have spoken to somebody who'd been through the system who could say, 'You know I've been through it and you're probably very confused'. Now, I could accept that coming from another patient but I'm damned if I could accept that coming from a doctor or a nurse." (Lester et al, 2006, pp 417-18, quoting former service user).

Paid employment can also help address wider issues of poverty and social isolation. However, employing service users in this way requires organisations to think about their own cultural environment. Service cultures that encourage involvement share a number of common characteristics, including a commitment to genuine partnerships between users and professionals and to the development of shared objectives. As the National Schizophrenia Fellowship (now Rethink) has observed:

> Everyone involved in the delivery of care ... should be treated as equal partners. Occasionally, some professionals may initially feel threatened by the involvement of service users and carers and if this is the case, then it is important that this issue is addressed so that all of the parties involved can work well together. (National Schizophrenia Fellowship, 1997, p 10)

The approach and value base of individual practitioners are also critical. Some professionals may find it difficult to view service users as experts. Although there is some evidence to suggest that mental health professionals are generally supportive of user involvement, there are also dissonances between expressed support and actual practice (Campbell, 2001). This may reflect resistance to the notion of sharing and transferring power to users, or a clash of professional 'scientific' and users' more 'social' ways of thinking and working (Summers, 2003). Above all, if involving experts by experience as co-workers remains a strategy largely enforced through policy directives, involvement of this 'hard to reach' group will continue to be largely tokenistic.

## Case study 2: user involvement for people who are homeless

Up to 4.3% of all current heads of household in England have experienced a period of homelessness in the past decade (Burrows et al, 1997). Recent statistics from Crisis suggest that there are over 162,000 households currently accepted as homeless by local authorities in England (www.crisis.org.uk, accessed 25 June 2006). According to the Office of the Deputy Prime Minister, Black and minority ethnic households represent 21% of those accepted as homeless. Homelessness represents social exclusion in its most extreme form. Homeless people are socially invisible and are often wary of authority (perhaps because up to 50% of rough sleepers have been in prison or a remand centre at some point in their life (SEU, 1998)). As a 'hard to reach' group, they also share many of the negative stereotypes associated with people with serious mental illness. Stereotypes of violence and unpredictability are common (Wright, 2002), though in fact rough sleepers are far more likely to be the recipients than perpetrators of violence (Fitzpatrick and Kennedy, 2000).

People who are homeless are 40 times more likely not to be registered with a GP than the general population (Crisis, 2002). Barriers to care are poorly researched, but limited work from a GP perspective suggests that lack of training, concerns over time costs and negative attitudes towards homeless people are significant issues (Lester and Bradley, 2001). Homeless people themselves report perceived reluctance from primary care teams and personal competing priorities as barriers to registration and care (Shiner, 1995). Homelessness has profound implications for health. Studies have shown that the mental and/or physical health of homeless people is considerably worse than that of the general population, with those at the extreme end of the housing spectrum suffering the poorest health (Bines, 1994; Warnes et al, 2003). Mental health problems are up to eight times more prevalent in homeless people (Bines, 1994). Perhaps the most overt example of health inequalities is that the life expectancy of a rough sleeper in England is only 42 years (Crisis, 1996).

Policy imperatives around user involvement for homeless people are limited (Crisis, 2003). The 2002 Homelessness Act has placed new duties on local authorities to carry out reviews and publish strategies to address and prevent homelessness in their areas that encompass users' views of services. User involvement may, nevertheless, seem low on a Maslowian hierarchy of needs (1954). However, if we focus, instead, on the notion of a hierarchy of involvement as reflected in Arnstein's ladder of participation (1969), applying boundaries to involvement is inappropriate. Homeless people have both a right and capacity to be involved. Indeed, the recent statement from the Homelessness Taskforce emphasises:

> ... the need to increase homeless people's control and extend their choices, particularly in relation to housing, employment, care and support services, and to achieve the effective participation of people affected by homelessness in the development of future policy, practice and service delivery. These objectives should be widely promoted and given practical effect in all activities directed at tackling homelessness. (Homelessness Taskforce, 2002, p 9)

### Examples of positive practice in encouraging user involvement for people who are homeless

There are a small number of largely voluntary sector organisations that are committed to inclusive approaches, and that work with people who are or have been homeless to set up and run projects to help themselves.

Groundswell (http://groundswell.org.uk) is a charity that since 1996 has been promoting practical solutions, that involve homeless people, to address homelessness and social exclusion. It is the organisation responsible for developing 'speak outs'. This methodology for encouraging user involvement was pioneered in Scotland by a group of homeless and ex-homeless people who wanted to provide a platform for homeless peoples' voices to be heard. They are community-based, people-led meetings that encourage everyone to 'have their say'. Key people such as planners and policy makers and the local media are actively encouraged to attend 'speak outs' and to listen and respond to concerns raised by homeless people.

Guidance on involving homeless people in 'speak outs' includes advice on practical issues such as venue (a community-based and safe setting), and on the importance of paying travel fares and including food at the event. 'Speak outs' are written up afterwards and copies sent to significant absentees, so people realise that their views have been taken seriously and are being considered.

'Speak outs' are valuable in raising self-esteem, which is, of itself, an important outcome. They can also highlight issues that have a more immediate effect on health equalities for people who are homeless. In recent years, they have helped to increase awareness of the new rights for people sleeping on the streets or in temporary accommodation to register and vote, meaning that homeless people have an opportunity to influence political decisions and play a fuller role as citizens.

## Conclusion

Creating and promoting greater exchange between those who provide and manage health services and communities and individuals who seek and receive services will create better tailoring of services to demand. More importantly, user involvement will inform and raise awareness of health concerns and is likely to be a key part of the process of moving to a 'fully engaged scenario' (Wanless, 2004). Current user involvement mechanisms, however, may promote tokenism and fail to understand and address the complexities of user involvement for people who are members of 'hard to reach' groups. Barriers to user involvement include a lack of information, time and money and user–professional power imbalances. For 'hard to reach' groups, there are additional problems of definition and the rarely acknowledged tensions created by seeking user views on the importance of involvement in the context of a disenfranchised existence. Involvement strategies are also over-reliant on the voluntary sector, who are commissioned to do participatory work by a public sector organisation, allowing such organisations to shift the responsibility and disengage from the process (Tritter et al, 2003). Such practices serve to reproduce and reinforce existing patterns of health inequality.

Meaningful user involvement should not be a one-off intervention or a discrete programme of work, but a much broader and more empowering way of working that affects every aspect of health provision. However, at the start of the new millennium, despite a plethora of policy reforms and pockets of good practice, it appears that a fundamental shift in the balance of power between users and professionals still remains to be achieved. User involvement is everyone's business but will require radical shifts in both theory and practice to succeed.

### Note

[1] We have adopted the term 'user involvement' throughout this chapter. The terminology continues to be contested and has included a range of terms, from citizen engagement through patient and public involvement. While 'user involvement' is also shunned by some, we feel it captures best the generic category of those patients, carers and

members of the public who may seek opportunities to comment on and shape the health services available in their community.

## References

Acheson, D. (1998) *Independent inquiry into inequalities in health*, London: The Stationery Office.

Anderson, W. and Florin, D. (2000) 'Consulting the public about the NHS', *BMJ*, vol 320, pp 1553-4.

Appleby, J., Harrison, A. and Devlin, N. (2003) *What is the real cost of more patient choice?*, London: Kings Fund.

Arnstein, S.R. (1969) 'A ladder of participation', *American Institute of Planners Journal*, vol 35, no 4, pp 216-24.

Bines, W. (1994) *The health of single homeless people*, York: Centre for Housing Policy, University of York.

Burrows, R., Pleace, N. and Quilgars, D. (1997) *Homelessness and social policy*, London and New York: Routledge.

Campbell, P. (2001) 'The role of users in psychiatric services in service development – influence not power', *Psychiatric Bulletin*, vol 25, no 3, pp 87-8.

Clark, M., Glasby, J. and Lester, H.E. (2004) 'User involvement in health care research', *Journal of Research Policy and Planning*, vol 22, no 2, pp 31-8.

Connolly, M. and Kelly, C. (2005) 'Lifestyle and physical health in schizophrenia', *Advances in Psychiatric Treatment*, vol 11, no 2, pp 125-32.

Cook, D. (2002) 'Consultation, for a change? Engaging users and communities in the policy process', *Social Policy and Administration*, vol 36, no 5, pp 516-31.

Crisis (1996) *Still dying for a home*, London: Crisis.

Crisis (2002) *Critical condition: Vulnerable single homeless people and access to GPs*, London: Crisis.

Crisis (2003) *Guide to models of delivering health services to homeless people*, London: Crisis.

Croft, S. and Beresford, P. (1993) 'User involvement, citizenship and social policy', *Critical Social Policy*, vol 9, no 26, pp 5-18.

Croft, S. and Beresford, P. (1995) 'Whose empowerment? Equalising the competing discourses in community care', in R. Jack (ed) *Empowerment in community care*, London: Chapman Hall, pp 59-73.

DH (Department of Health) (1991) *The patient's charter*, London: HMSO.

DH (1992) *The health of the nation*, London: The Stationery Office.

DH (1994) *Working in partnership: a collaborative approach to care: Report of the mental health nursing review*, London: HMSO.

DH (1995) *Building bridges: A guide to the arrangements for interagency working for the care and protection of severely disabled people*, London: DH.

DH (2000) *The NHS Plan: A plan for investment, a plan for reform*, London: The Stationery Office.

DH (2001) *The report of the public inquiry into children's heart surgery at the Bristol Royal Infirmary 1984–1995: Learning from Bristol*, Cm 5207, London: HMSO.

DH (2002a) *Addressing inequalities – reaching 'hard to reach' group. National Service Frameworks. A practical aid to implementation in primary care*, London: DH.

DH (2002b) *The government's vision for mental health care*, London: DH.

DH (2003a) *Building on the best: Choice, responsiveness and equity in the NHS*, Cm 6079, London: The Stationery Office.

DH (2003b) *Strengthening accountability: Involving patients and the public – policy guidance, Section 11 of the Health and Social Care Act 2001*, London: DH.

DH (2003c) *Mental health policy implementation guide: Support, time and recovery workers*, London: DH.

DH (2005) *Creating a patient-led NHS: Delivering the NHS improvement plan*, London: DH.

DH (2006a) *A stronger local voice: A framework for creating a stronger local voice in the development of health and social care services*, London: DH.

DH (2006b) *The government's response to 'A stronger local voice'*, London: DH.

Doherty, P., Stott, A. and Kinder, K. (2004) *Delivering services to hard to reach families in On Track areas: Definition, consultation and needs assessment*, Home Office Development and Practice Report 15, London: Research, Development and Statistics Directorate, Home Office.

Edmans, T. and Taket, A. (2001) 'Community-led regeneration – experiences from London', Paper presented to the Irish Social Policy Association, Dublin, July.

Faugier, J. and Sargeant, M. (1997) 'Sampling "hard to reach" populations', *Journal of Advanced Nursing*, vol 26, no 4, pp 790-7.

Feldberg, G. and Vipond, R. (1999) 'The virus of consumerism', in D. Drache and T. Sullivan (eds) *Health reform: Public success, private failure*, London: Routledge, pp 448-64.

Fitzpatrick, S. and Kennedy, C. (2000) *Getting by: Begging, rough sleeping and* The Big Issue *in Glasgow and Edinburgh*, Bristol: The Policy Press.

Ford, R., Durcan, G., Warner, L., Hardy, P. and Muijen, M. (1998) 'One day survey by the Mental Health Act Commission of acute adult psychiatric inpatient wards in England and Wales', *BMJ*, vol 317, pp 1279-83.

Freedland, J. (1998) 'Out of the bin and glad to be mad', *The Guardian*, 21 January.

Homelessness Taskforce (2002) *Homelessness: An action plan for prevention and effective response. Report from the Homelessness Taskforce to Scottish ministers*, Edinburgh: Scottish Executive.

HSE (Health and Safety Executive) (2004) *Successful interventions with 'hard to reach' groups*, London: HSE.

Involve (2003) *Strategic plan 2003-2006: Creating the expert resource*, Eastleigh: Involve.

Jewesbury, I. (1998) *Risks and rights: Mentally disordered offenders and public protection*, London: Nacro.

Jones, J. and Newburn, T. (2001) *The policing and reducing crime unit*, Police Research Series Paper 138, London: Home Office.

Lester, H.E. and Bradley, C.P. (2001) 'Barriers to primary health care for homeless people – the general practitioner perspective', *European Journal of General Practice*, vol 7, pp 6-12.

Lester, H.E., Tait, L., England, E. and Tritter J.Q. (2006) 'Patient involvement in primary care mental health: a focus group study', *British Journal of General Practice*, vol 56, no 527, pp 415-22.

Lester, H.E., Tritter, J.Q. and Sorohan, H. (2005) 'Patients' and health professionals' views on primary care for people with serious mental illness: focus group study', *BMJ*, vol 330, pp 1122-8.

Madison, J. (1961[1787]) 'The utility of the union as a safeguard against domestic faction and insurrection', in A. Hamilton, J. Madison and J. Jay (1961[1788]) *The Federalist Papers*, London: New English Library.

Marder, S.R., Essock, S.M., Miller, A.L., Buchanan, R.W., Casey, D.E., Davis, J.M., Kane, J.M., Lieberman, J.A., Schooler, N.R., Covell, N., Stroup, S., Weissman, E.M., Wirshing, D.A., Hall, C.S., Pogach, L., Pi-Sunyer, X., Bigger, J.T., Jr., Friedman, A., Kleinberg, D., Yevich, S.J., Davis, B. and Shon, S. (2004) 'Physical health monitoring of patients with schizophrenia', *American Journal of Psychiatry*, vol 161, no 8, pp 1334-49.

Maslow, A.H. (1954) *Motivation and personality*, New York, NY: Harper and Row.

McCabe, A. and Ford, C. (2001) *Redressing the balance: Crime and mental health*, Manchester: UK Public Health Association.

Mukherjee, S., Decina, P., Bocola, V., Saraceni, F. and Scapicchio, P.L. (1996) 'Diabetes mellitus in schizophrenic patients', *Comprehensive Psychiatry*, vol 37, no 1, pp 68-73.

National Schizophrenia Fellowship (1997) *How to involve users and carers in planning, running and monitoring care services and curriculum development*, Kingston-upon-Thames: National Schizophrenia Fellowship.

NHS Management Executive (1992) *Local voices: The views of local people in purchasing for health*, Leeds: NHS Management Executive.

ODPM (Office of the Deputy Prime Minister) (2004) *Mental health and social exclusion*, Social Exclusion Unit Report, London: ODPM.

ONS (Office for National Statistics) (2002) *Labour Force Survey*, London: ONS.

Perkins, R., Choy, D. and Davidson, B. (1999) *Pathfinder user employment programme: Progress report*, London: Pathfinder Mental Health Trust.

Poxton, R. (2003) 'What makes effective partnerships between health and social care?', in J. Glasby and E. Peck (eds) *Care trusts: Partnership working in action*, Abingdon: Radcliffe Medical Press.

Sayce, L. (1997) 'Stigma and social exclusion: top priorities for mental health professionals', *Eurohealth*, vol 3, no 3, pp 5-7.

Sayce, L. (1999) 'High time for justice', *Nursing Times*, vol 95, no 9, pp 64-6.

Sayce, L. (2000) *From psychiatric patient to citizen: Overcoming discrimination and social exclusion*, Basingstoke: Palgrave.

Sayce, L. (2001) 'Social inclusion and mental health', *Psychiatric Bulletin*, vol 25, no 4, pp 121-3.

Sayce, L. and Morris, D. (1999) *Outsiders coming in? Achieving social inclusion for people with mental health problems*, London: Mind Publications.

SEU (Social Exclusion Unit) (1998) *Rough sleeping*, London: SEU.

Shiner, M. (1995) 'Adding insult to injury: homelessness and health service use', *Sociology of Health and Illness*, vol 17, no 4, pp 525-49.

Singleton, N., Bumpstead, R., O'Brien, M., Lee, A. and Meltzer, H. (2001) *Psychiatric morbidity among adults living in private households 2000*, London: The Stationery Office.

Summers, A. (2003) 'Involving users in the development of mental health services: a study of psychiatrists' views', *Journal of Mental Health*, vol 12, no 2, pp 161-74.

Taylor, P.J. and Gunn, J. (1999) 'Homicides by people with mental illness: myth and reality', *British Journal of Psychiatry*, vol 174, no 1, pp 9-14.

Tritter, J. and Macallum, A. (2006) 'The snakes and ladders of user involvement: moving beyond Arnstein', *Health Policy*, vol 76, no 2, pp 156-68.

Tritter, J. Daykin, N., Sanidas, M., Barley, V., Evans, S., McNeill, J., Palmer, N., Rimmer, J. and Turton, P. (2003) 'Divided care and the third way: user involvement in statutory and voluntary sector cancer services', *Sociology of Health and Illness*, vol 25, no 5, pp 429-56.

Wallcraft, J. and Bryant, M. (2003) *The mental health service users movement in England*, London: Sainsbury Centre for Mental Health.

Wanless, D. (2004) *Securing good health for the whole population. Final report*, London: HMSO (www.hm-treasury.gov.uk/consultations_and_legislation/wanless/consult_wanless04_final.cfm).

Warnes, T., Crane, M., Whitehead, N. and Fu, R. (2003) *Homelessness factfile*, London: Crisis.

Wilkinson, R.G. (1996) *Unhealthy societies: The afflictions of inequality*, London: Routledge.

Wright, N. (2002) *Homelessness: A primary care response*, London: Royal College of General Practitioners.

# ELEVEN

# Gilding the ghetto again? Community development approaches to tackling health inequalities

*Mick Carpenter*

## Introduction

The publication of the Acheson Report (Acheson, 1998) ended nearly two decades of political denial of health inequalities following the publication of the 1980 Black Report (Townsend et al, 1992). The key policy issue since 1997 has been whether New Labour is making progress in tackling health inequalities, including whether the government's initial commitment to tackling them has strengthened or diminished since Acheson. Since much assessment has sought to provide a bird's-eye view of the adequacy of macro-level policies, this chapter seeks to provide a complementary 'worm's-eye' view of the actual and potential role of local initiatives, particularly those informed by 'broad' community development principles.

The chapter starts by revisiting broad alternative macro-level strategies for tackling health inequalities, suggesting that insufficient attention has been given to the question of how they might intersect with micro-level interventions, which has often been implied rather than explicitly stated. The fundamental point made is that contested macro-level strategies are linked to parallel 'broader' and 'narrower' community development discourses. The implications of this are followed through in the remainder of the chapter. The danger identified is that New Labour has been pursuing a 'narrower' approach to community development that, despite some improvements on such approaches in the past, still tends to repeat the mistakes of the 1960s and '70s, when radical critics accused governments of merely seeking to 'gild the ghetto' rather than tackling external structural causes (Craig, 1989). After a brief conceptual review of the origins of community development approaches to health, New Labour's 'turn to the community' is critically assessed in relation to the possibilities and limitations of Area-based Initiatives (ABIs). This leads into a discussion of questions of evidence related to political and scientific evaluation issues, and the necessarily uncertain impact of localised initiatives on health inequalities. My overall conclusion is that broader community development strategies have an integral part to play in developing a new synthesis between 'top-down' structuralist approaches and 'bottom-up' participative approaches to tackling health inequalities.

## Community development and health inequalities policy discourses

The relationship between community development strategies and health inequalities is complex. Originally community development was conceived narrowly in terms of harnessing local 'self-help' to tackle poverty independently of the state. However, critiques of this traditional model advocated connecting it to broader questions of politics, empowerment and social justice, in which health gained greater prominence as a feature of community disadvantage. This broader approach received endorsement in health policy through the World Health Organization (WHO) 1986 Ottawa Charter, discussed later in this chapter. 'Best practice' definitions of community development now routinely articulate a broader approach. For example, a widely accepted definition in the UK is that of Community Development Exchange, which argues that it is centrally informed by values and commitments, and defines it as:

> ... building active and sustainable communities based on
> social justice and mutual respect. It is about changing power
> structures to remove the barriers that prevent people from
> participating in the issues that affect their lives. (CDX,
> 2006)

An influential Canadian definition also emphasises the importance of principles and values such as participation and inclusion. It envisages community development as a participative 'grassroots process' involving:

> ... the planned evolution of all aspects of community well-
> being (economic, social, environmental and cultural). It is
> a process whereby community members come together to
> take collective action and generate solutions to common

problems.... The primary outcome of community
development is improved quality of life. (Flank and Smith,
1999, p 6)

Health is something in these models that can be seen potentially as a
*resource* for community development, but more importantly as a key
*outcome*. It is noteworthy that these broad definitions do not equate
community development with community self-reliance, though nearly
all endorse 'capacity building', which is seen as action to 'enable' and
strengthen a community's skills and abilities, including the willingness
and ability to participate (Flank and Smith, 1999, p 10). In the context of
this chapter, it would mean embedding in the routines and structures of
community life institutions and practices that enhance health and well-
being, as well as knowledge and skills relevant to health. In a narrow
sense, 'capacity building' *could* be and often is equated with community
self-reliance, but can and *should* also link to broader questions about
the role of economic forces and government action in facilitating or
negating this process.

In connecting these issues to health inequalities policies, one problem
is that policy debates are often polarised between what, for shorthand
purposes, can be called 'macro-structural' and 'local agency'-focused
approaches. There are significant internal debates within the former
about whether to target relative or absolute poverty, and whether
economic redistribution or a redistribution of social and economic
power is the main objective (for example, Wilkinson, 1996; Lynch, et
al, 2000). However, all endorse what the 1998 Acheson Report calls
the 'socioeconomic model', which focuses on the need to take strong
societal-level action. There is a focus on tackling the 'health gradient'
across the social scale, rather than simply ameliorating the economic
status and health condition of the worst off. There is understandable
suspicion of the 'local agency' approach associated with New Labour
with its 'supply-side' preference for changing the poorest individuals and
communities, and avoidance of taking strong governmental action to
tackle structural inequality (see also Chapter Three of this volume). This
critique, arguably, often leads to a top-down and paternalistic approach.
Since the factors influencing health are typically seen as largely beyond
individual or local community control, there is an under-emphasis on
the role that local agency could play. Thus, the vast majority of the 39
recommendations made by the Acheson Report proposed national
action. Only the last one, in passing, briefly endorsed the need for
local partnerships between local statutory agencies, the voluntary and

private sector and local people, and community development is not mentioned anywhere in the report.

In this regard, it is important to identify the positives associated with New Labour's rediscovery of the community, against Thatcher's assertion to *Woman's Own* in 1987 that 'there is no such thing as society'. In asserting that poverty and well-being are a community responsibility, New Labour has also taken some lessons from the failed community initiatives of the past. There is recognition of the need to develop participative approaches that engage with and involve local communities most affected by health inequalities, tackling problems in collaborative ways. The government also claims that it is taking broader action to tackle poverty, unemployment and other issues at central level. However, while making token gestures in the direction of broader definitions of community development and capacity building, in reality a much narrower version is being implemented that is focused on limited support to promote community self-reliance. Official enthusiasm for community development is usually channelled through ABIs leading to a primary focus almost exclusively on those at the bottom to the exclusion of the health gradient as a whole. In addition, there have often been excessive expectations of what local communities can achieve within short-term funding regimes, thus potentially setting initiatives up for failure.

Much of the recent emphasis on local capacity building, generally and in relation to health, has been influenced by the work of Putnam (2000), which focuses on the role of 'social capital' or the strengthening of social networks in ways that arguably underplay the role of material pressures. This is symptomatic of a failure of New Labour policies to tackle health inequalities by targeting inequality itself. This derives from a supply-side political economy, strongly oriented towards welfare to work, aiming primarily to reinforce people's ability to deal with competitive forces rather than offering significant protection against them. Increasingly, however, the emphasis in the early days of New Labour on community development shifted towards a more medicalised emphasis on changing individual lifestyle to combat epidemiologically identified 'risk factors', particularly in relation to smoking, alcohol, drugs, diet and exercise (DH, 2004). There has thus been an increasing shift in emphasis from local community to individual agency. Empowerment or 'agency' in this context means, as the public health White Paper puts it, being enabled to make 'healthy choices'. These, however, tend to be externally prescribed in terms of a hierarchical rational choice model (for a critique of which, see Archer and Tritter, 2000). This is underlined by the resort to health 'trainers' to transmit medicalised commands (DH, 2004; see also Chapters Three and Nine of this volume).

The message of this chapter, developed further in the conclusion, is that adoption of a broader model of community development and capacity building can and needs to be synthesised with a strong structuralist approach. This cannot be achieved if it is ignored or simply dismissed as a New Labour diversionary tactic. Without exaggerating the possibilities, it is possible to identify ways in which local action based on community development principles can empower disadvantaged communities and address the problems that beset them. Such a 'multilevel strategy' can be facilitated through consideration of the renowned Dahlgren-Whitehead 'layers of influence' model, as adapted by the UK Public Health Association (2006), to give some prominence to local and neighbourhood influences.

## Top-down and bottom-up tensions in community development

While there is a need for a synthesis of top-down and bottom-up approaches, the potential tensions between them must also be acknowledged. This requires some consideration of the historical context if the wheel is not to be reinvented. As already mentioned, New Labour showed some awareness of these issues after 1997. The government recognised that token gestures to community involvement that were common in the past were a prime reason for the failure of previous ABIs, and there was a need to grant communities real powers, with significant resources, over a significant time period. In short, New Labour has seemingly acknowledged that empowerment of communities, combined with joined-up government at the local level, needs to be central to strategies to tackle neighbourhood disadvantage. Thus in the National Strategy for Neighbourhood Renewal in 2001 (Cabinet Office, 2001), health was recognised alongside issues such as low income, unemployment, housing and educational disadvantage, crime and environmental degradation to be a significant feature of community disadvantage.

While community development has a long history in Britain, it is only relatively recently that health has been articulated as a significant objective within it. The general roots of community development were conservative and top-down in the efforts by charities and elite reformers in the late 19th century to 'remoralise' the poor and promote 'self-help' (Craig, 1989). For this reason, Fabian socialist reformers largely rejected it in favour of nationally based, state collectivist solutions, and the Black and Acheson Reports are firmly situated in this tradition. While the welfare state saw a decline in community and voluntary action, it was revived in the 1960s through top-down efforts to find solutions to growing urban problems, and also as part of a bottom-up, collectivist, self-help challenge to the professionalised welfare state. The tension between these elements remains within New Labour approaches. Current developments were foreshadowed in the 1970s and ' 80s in efforts by some left-wing Labour councils to pioneer new decentralised and participative approaches to local planning and delivery of public services. Social movements around race, gender, sexuality and disability often foregrounded health issues by challenging the medical model, and articulating a social model linking personal and structural transformation.

Thus it would be a mistake to believe that nothing happened in the field of health inequalities for two decades after the Conservative government suppressed the Black Report in the 1980s. Since it was the only way forward, the report unintentionally stimulated local experiments of one kind or another. This trend was reinforced by the landmark WHO (1981) Health for All by the Year 2000 Strategy, which shifted attention 'upstream' towards non-medical means of promoting health, despite or even because of the lack of official encouragement from Conservative governments that regarded it as too socialistic. Radical 'community medicine' professionals in a range of local areas sought to develop alliances with disadvantaged and oppressed communities that perhaps later lost their missionary zeal when they become mainstreamed within local bureaucracies. The WHO Healthy Cities initiatives in 1987 gave impetus to public health professionals in a number of areas in the UK to take action in broad holistic, preventive and participative ways, with Camden, Liverpool and Belfast being WHO-designated sites. Other cities, such as Sheffield, sought to develop local Health for All strategies (Smithies and Webster, 1998, pp 12-13). A key development was the shift from a health education to a health promotion discourse, stimulated by the WHO 1986 Ottawa Charter's explicit advocacy of a community development approach that:

> ... draws on existing human and material resources in the community to enhance self-help and social support, and to develop flexible systems for strengthening public participation in and direction of health matters. This requires full and continuous access to information, learning opportunities for health, as well as funding support. (WHO, 1986, p 3)

By the early 1990s, with the departure of Thatcher, even under a Conservative government ideological shifts started to occur, which, among other things, led to more inclusive urban regeneration programmes and permission to talk about health 'variations' if not inequalities. Efforts to encourage 'local voices' and 'healthy alliances' received more official encouragement through the 1993 White Paper, *The health of the nation* (Smithies and Webster, 1998, pp 24-6, 31). These shifts were consolidated by New Labour policies, to which the chapter now turns.

## New Labour, the community and health inequalities

One of the claims made in the name of New Labour is that it has led to the adoption of a distinct 'Third Way' between classic social democracy and the free market. As Driver and Martell (2000) among others have pointed out, not everything is in fact 'new'. For example, we have seen how a reliance on ABIs and efforts to pioneer new forms of local governance started to develop under 'Old' Labour. Driver and Martell also point out that a variety of 'Third Ways' have contested the field, with some arguing for greater emphasis on government intervention and redistributive measures. However, rather than reduce inequality, New Labour's anti-poverty strategy has sought to lift the floor for poor people, through measures that increase the attractiveness of paid work through a minimum wage and tax credits, and welfare-to-work schemes that help enhance people's employability (see also Chapter Five of this volume). The income of those reliant on state benefits has fallen behind, as benefits continue to be uprated in line with prices rather than earnings. This general strategy has been combined with ABIs of one kind or another to tackle the spatial dimensions of poverty, notably New Deal for Communities (NDC), Sure Start and other initiatives channelled through Local Strategic Partnerships (LSPs). However, the assumptions are often that there is no need to reduce inequality as such, which is seen as functional for a dynamic and open economy.

In this regard, Levitas (1998, ch 3) has identified a number of discourses around poverty and social policy: 'RED', a redistributionist discourse, linked to a structural analysis; 'MUD', a moral underclass discourse, linked to a cultural-behavioural deficit model; and 'SID' a social integrationist discourse, strongly associated with encouraging participation in paid employment. Since 1997, New Labour's approach to poverty and health inequality has largely focused on MUD and SID. However, more collectivist voices within New Labour have argued for RED, or lowering the ceiling as well as raising the floor, and this would be consistent with tackling the health gradient as a whole. This is essentially the perspective of the Acheson Report, though perhaps not as explicitly articulated as it might be. This indicates tensions between it and mainstream New Labour approaches to health inequalities, which have become more apparent with the publication of the 2004 public health White Paper (DH, 2004).

The roots of this New Labour caution lie in the frequently stated belief in the need to adapt to rather than control capitalist globalisation through an open economy and flexible labour markets. The first priority is given to maintaining a stable currency and low inflation, which includes a reluctance to intervene in ways that might dent confidence in Britain as a place to invest. This is the constraining framework within which criticisms of unbridled Thatcherite individualism and support for the notions of 'community' are made. However, it also has the statism of traditional social democracy in its sights through advocacy of an 'enabling' state that strengthens rather than replaces people's own efforts. Thus, Tony Blair argued in 2002 that: 'The state can sometimes become part of the problem, by smothering the enthusiasm of its citizens ... Responsive public services are part of the solution. We also need to do more to give power directly to citizens ... Communities that are inter-connected are healthier' (Blair, 2002, p 10).

There is undoubtedly substantial evidence of the importance of social networks and 'trust'-based relationships to health (for example, Kawachi et al, 2004). This evidence supports a holistic view of health and arguments that we 'need' social connectedness as well as individual autonomy (Doyal and Gough, 1991). Yet New Labour's approach to community development, while paying lip service to collective empowerment, has predominantly endorsed more conservative approaches based on communitarian US thinkers such as Amitai Etzioni and Robert Putnam (Fremeaux, 2005). These focus on promoting self-reliant 'capacity building' and even community social control. This can lead to exaggerated expectations of what can be achieved simply by strengthening social networks by enhancing 'social capital'. This can often lead to 'deficit' models of local communities that are seen as lacking these characteristics.

The reliance on local effort to bring about change is embedded in initiatives like NDCs, Sure Start and LSPs, which are expected to meet a range of targets imposed on them from above by central government, as well as engaging in time-consuming performance management procedures. The key health inequalities targets are top-down, medically defined targets centred on reducing infant mortality and raising life expectancy. They can potentially divert attention away from the need, identified by nearly all authorities as desirable and effective practice in community health promotion, to start from community-defined health issues and problems (for example, Taylor, 2003). There is a need also to recognise that communities are made up of diverse voices and interests by age, gender and ethnicity that may not be always fully represented by those 'usual suspects' who actively participate in community initiatives (Gilchrist, 2003; Taylor, 2003; see also Chapter Ten of this volume).

The health inequalities targets established as a result of the Treasury's cross-cutting review (HM Treasury and DH, 2002) have been of two kinds in health, as elsewhere in social policy. They have either sought to establish minimum standards, 'floor targets', often compared with the approach taken by the national minimum wage, or else they have sought to close gaps between disadvantaged groups and the average. In both cases, they underline the fact that New Labour has not been seeking to achieve greater equality across the social scale between the least and most disadvantaged social groups (see Chapter Three of this volume). This is informed by the notion that there is just a problem 'at the bottom' in the post-industrial 'knowledge' society that can largely be solved by integrating problem people into the mainstream economy. This is open to the challenge that there is a general issue of inequality that needs tackling. This has been highlighted in terms of a growing trend towards a dual or 'hourglass' economy, characterised by increasing polarisation between a growing number of insecure and poorly paid jobs at the base and an expanded number of well-paid jobs at the top (Nolan, 2004). A dual economy generates spatial inequalities that are reflected in an overheated South East, where housing costs act as a bar to participation in low-paid service work, and in economic decline in significant parts of the Midlands, the North, Scotland, Wales and Northern Ireland. People from minority ethnic groups, as well as growing numbers of new migrant communities, are concentrated in many of the areas worst affected. What this analysis indicates is that if health inequalities are to be adequately addressed, there is a need not only to target deep-seated social inequalities through redistributive measures, but also to implement 'upstream' interventions in the underlying political economic processes that generate them. In 'critical realist' terms, these would be seen as the 'generative mechanisms' (Bhaskar, 1978).

While broader approaches to community development can accommodate these structural issues, centrist or communitarian approaches tend to isolate the influence of lifestyle and social networks from the broader contexts in which they are embedded. Deficits in 'social capital' are therefore not seen as a reflection but a prime cause of social disadvantage. By contrast, Law and Mooney (2006) argue that poverty and capitalist change have a destructive effect on social networks. While it cannot be denied that class-related patterns of consumption like smoking are important, the mistake is not to see these as embedded in unequal social relations, and portray them as largely matters of individual or cultural agency (see also Chapter Nine of this volume). Thus it is well established that efforts to target individual lifestyles widen health inequalities, as advice is taken up more by high-income groups (Carlisle, 2001; Wilkinson and Marmot, 2003). Recently, promising efforts have been made to link structural inequality and social network analysis within a 'structure-agency' paradigm (Szreter and Woolcock, 2004). While promising, some critics argue that they still under-emphasise the role of structural contexts and question the use of 'social capital' as a way of understanding the influence of social networks (Moore et al, 2006). Despite these problems, this emerging debate shows that it may be possible to overcome the polarisation between macro-structural and local agency approaches, creating theoretical and policy–practice bridges between them.

## Evaluating local health inequalities policies: tool of the centre or in the vanguard of change?

The Acheson Report made much of the need for central government to take concerted upstream action on 'healthy public policy' to prevent downstream health inequalities. However, the reliance on local agency and fears, for reasons already discussed, of alienating business interests mean that there have at best been only modest moves in these directions. A prime and important example of this is government action to tackle smoking in public places, where the initial proposed legislation, exempting pubs and clubs that did not serve food, could have worsened health inequalities. A universal ban emerged, somewhat against the odds, only after pressure from a 'healthy alliance' of pressure groups, health professionals, the trade union movement and individual politicians. This was 'evidence based' in that the pressure for a ban mounted as a result of increasingly convincing evidence of the dangers of passive smoking. There were also workable examples to draw on from Ireland and elsewhere, and a devolved Scottish Parliament increased the pressure on the rest of the UK by legislating for a total ban. Legislation by the UK Parliament for a total ban came about partly because campaigners were able to achieve a shift in public discourse from concerns about interfering with individual freedom to recognition, reinforced by European legislation, of a need to protect the health and safety rights of workers in bars and the hospitality industry. The government U-turn in favour of a total ban was also influenced by fears that local action might go further than national legislation, as Liverpool and London councils were threatening to promote their own bans in the House of Lords (Arnott and Willmore, 2006; see also Chapter Nine for further discussion of the issues of controlling smoking behaviour).

This is just one example of how local action, in combination with social movements, can combine to put interests hostile to health on the defensive and start to force the hand of national government. Another health-related example, which has yet to bear wider fruit, is the introduction by the Mayor of London, Ken Livingstone, of a traffic congestion charge in central London, which has been argued to have equitable as well as general benefits to health and well-being (Clark, 2003). This demonstrates, in an era when the public sector is under challenge, that it is possible to develop effective administrative instruments that start to tackle some of our most deeply embedded health and environmental issues. Thus the relationship between evidence and action is a question not simply of implementing 'what works', but also of devising imaginative policy instruments on the one hand and, crucially, finding the political means to implement them on the other. Health inequalities research has perhaps got too bogged down in debates about causes and pathways, and there is a greater need to link their implications to case study analyses of political processes and administrative means (Exworthy et al, 2006).

In this regard, a key issue identified by this chapter is the fact that macro-structural approaches often give too little acknowledgement of the potential of community development, while narrow conceptions of 'capacity building' place excessive faith on the possibilities of community self-reliance. A broader and more radical approach, such as that developed by Ledwith (2005), drawing on feminism and the work of Paulo Freire (1986), offers a way of providing linkages between central and local interventions, aligning it with the empowerment and social change principles of the WHO Ottawa Charter. Such an approach, like the examples just given, shows how action from 'below' can help to bring about the wider changes also needed from 'above'. The debate about means has become pressing in the context of the establishment of local health inequalities targets from 2002 (Sassi, 2005). Yet it also needs to be said that some health policies introduced by central government seem to work in counter directions. Thus, shifts to the market and patient choice are likely to empower middle-class health users most, widening access inequalities (see also Chapter Nine). The White Paper on public health (DH, 2004) undoubtedly identified health inequalities as a priority, and drew attention to the wider actions that local agencies, including local authorities, could undertake to promote health. However, it shifted the weight of policy attention towards changing individual lifestyles and away from tackling structural issues and community capacity building.

In terms of the issues raised by this chapter, it seems a pity that Health Action Zones (HAZs) were only a brief experiment of the years immediately after the 1997 election of New Labour, with hardly any time to flourish before being disbanded. Admittedly, they gave way to broader-based, larger-scale ABIs like NDCs, and setting up LSPs to take coordinated and participative local action to tackle a range of inequalities, including employment, housing, education and crime, as well as health. The conclusion of members of HAZ projects was that they had not had sufficient time to make more than a minimal impact on health inequalities (HDA, 2004a). Arguably one of the most significant contributions made by HAZs was to shift the question of evaluation on to a new footing through advocacy of 'theory-led' or 'realistic' evaluation methods. These recognise the importance of linking causal mechanisms to project objectives through 'theories of change' that take account of community set agendas, and, in testing them out, take account of the influence of wider contexts, participative relations and partnership effects (Pawson and Tilley, 1997; Hills, 2004; Barnes et al, 2005). Realistic evaluation focuses on both process and outcomes, and is based on a critique of the appropriateness of quasi-experimental methods that manipulate one or two variables, though they still have their defenders. However, it is possible to develop 'intermediate' indicators of health change, including the creation of effective local partnership relationships, which if sustained over time could plausibly lead to health gain. The framework developed by Nutbeam (1998) offers a range of health promotion outcomes, including health literacy, social mobilisation and relevant public policies, within which local health inequalities strategies could be assessed. This framework can operate at a range of levels. It has been used in evaluating a range of local health projects, and also informs the European Union's public health strategy.

One of the emerging evaluation lessons is that projects need time, and that people need to be tracked over a prolonged period. In practice, however, it is common to judge success by short-term change, for example, if someone gets employment with 13 weeks or stops smoking after four weeks. Awareness of complexity issues would also encourage 'realism' in the sense of encouraging modesty about claims as to what works, since, as well as broader context effects, local people may be exposed to a range of interventions rather than just the one being tested. These considerations, relevant to a broader community development approach, are not always appreciated by local and national politicians and decision makers in agencies, who often operate with 'simple' notions of 'what works', and expect 'hard' data in the short term to proclaim the success of what they do (Coote et al, 2004; Judge and Bauld, 2006). For example, a local initiative in Coventry that resulted in a reduction in the number of teenage pregnancies in one year was proclaimed a success by central government. The following year, however, the rate of teenage pregnancies had reverted to what it had been before the initiative began. This suggests a need to wait a number of years before assessing whether fluctuating trends indicate progress or not. Top-down pressure to deliver on predetermined short-term targets also militates against local ownership and empowerment, which may be counterproductive.

Certainly, since 1997 there has been a broad range of interventions that have either directly or indirectly targeted health. Following the *Choosing health* White Paper (DH, 2004), local government was identified as having a leadership role to play, consistent with the Acheson Report's emphasis on the importance of non-medical interventions. This has been associated with the development of initiatives such as 'Beacon Councils', which are pioneering a range of 'model' interventions, and a Communities for Health programme (Municipal Journal, 2005). Since the 2001 Health and Social Care Act, local authorities have been empowered to set up Health Scrutiny Committees and many have sought to tackle health inequalities. Examples include the London Borough of Camden, which has examined the health impacts of housing repairs, while other areas have focused on particular groups' needs, such as men's health in Stockport and Pakistani women in Sandwell, while Greenwich looked at the impact of the local authority as a whole on health inequalities (HDA, 2004b). After 2002, Primary Care Trusts (PCTs) have been required to use Health Equity Audits (HEAs) to inform service planning and their partnership working with other local agencies, which can also be used for assessing the needs of minority ethnic groups (HDA, 2005). From 2006, the most important local initiatives, including partnership work through LSPs, will be channelled through Local Area Agreements (LAAs). These allow for some flexibility in local target setting, with financial rewards for good performance. Health Impactment Assessment (HIA) is a policy tool that can be used to develop local healthier and equitable public policies. Consistent with community development aims, some practitioners have often sought to work in participative ways. Resort to HIA, however, is currently patchy (www.hiagateway.org.uk).

The spread of these activities undoubtedly helps to mainstream action on health inequalities within a wider local context than ABIs, but they add to the multiplicity of initiatives that succeed one another. In 2005, the government produced a manual of advice that is helpful, if in a rather 'top-down' way, in relation to government policies, and scanning it shows the bewildering multiplicity of relevant local initiatives (ODPM, 2005). As indicated above, there is as yet a lack of robust evidence on their effects, and it has been easier to evaluate processes than outcomes. On the whole, it can be seen that projects are variously seeking to provide material support, promote 'healthy' lifestyles, improve access to secondary care, promote general well-being, build community capacity, or enhance life skills. Increasingly, in Coventry as elsewhere, health messages are being transmitted through 'peer' or link workers recruited from disadvantaged communities. However, almost universally, while they are seeking and are sometimes demonstrably liberating agency with positive empowering and health effects, they are doing so *within* structures and have limited transformative effects (see Chapter Eight for further comment on food-based initiatives).

There are a range of possible impacts on health, defined by objective or subjective criteria, which might range from neutral effects, through preventing a worsening of health, to positive health gain. The studies so far conducted indicate that, though there is some potential for gain, neighbourhood regeneration can also involve substantial change that may be experienced as disruption. In the longer term, for example, housing improvements can lead to health gain, but displacement or inconvenience of residents can have short-term negative effects. Improved housing may also be more costly and this can have direct income effects and indirect psychosocial effects through worry about making ends meet (Ambrose, 2001). A review of available evidence from nine major UK ABIs concluded that evaluation of outcomes as opposed to outputs was uncommon. There was evidence of some small improvements to health and associated indicators such as employment and education, but also some negative results (Thomson et al, 2006). Another review by Curtis and colleagues (2002) found similar results, and pointed out that the damage already done by deprivation and inequality may take some considerable time to ameliorate or reverse, if at all.

Empowerment and involvement are often regarded as having positive health effects, and indeed the author's work in Coventry and wider research evidence confirms that people report that involvement in community projects has been beneficial for their health and well-being in a variety of ways. However, available research also shows a downside. The considerable demands that unpaid community participation makes can be exhausting, and even lead to burn-out (Kagan, 2006). Such costs reinforce concerns that the government's strategy may be placing too much responsibility on people from disadvantaged communities to turn things around themselves, and more weight needs to be put on intervening 'upstream' at the source of the problem, and to improve mainstream public services for disadvantaged people. It should not be assumed that meeting government targets of improved life expectancy is necessarily the highest priority for people struggling with day-to-day survival. A holistic approach focused on improving disadvantaged and excluded people's material and social well-being in a society with ample economic resources can be justified on the grounds of social justice. Though it is likely to provide many tangible health benefits, taking action should not be conditional on proving indisputably that it will help meet government targets.

## Conclusion: top down meets bottom up?

This chapter has identified many positives features associated with the growth of local action to tackle health inequalities. It has also pointed to some critical issues. These include the need to develop more robust models of empowerment and holistic evaluation models that link local intervention to broader social change, show the complexities involved in change processes, and take account of community-defined priorities. It is too early to characterise New Labour initiatives as simply 'gilding the ghetto' again, as its policies may start to narrow health inequalities in time. However, this will be achieved not only by targeted initiatives, but also by the whole range of government policies. In this regard, there remains a disparity between the evidence of a health gradient spanning society, and a range of policies that are primarily aimed at improving the position of the most severely disadvantaged groups, with excessive reliance on ABIs. There is also a disparity between a liberalised economy with increasingly polarised rich and poor, with regional, local and neighbourhood effects, and the failure of governments to intervene to correct them. While appearing to endorse the empowerment of communities, the government continues to impose predetermined targets on them. In doing so, it has been better at prescribing healthy public policy responsibilities for others than taking concerted action in its own back yard.

This chapter has highlighted the vital though necessarily uncertain effects of local action to promote health and well-being and tackle health inequalities. It has thus shown some of the complexities involved in identifying what kind of evidence matters and for whom in evidence-based policy and practice. It has argued for a broader rather than a narrower conception of community development, principally on the grounds of social justice, from which its presumed health benefits cannot be separated. Above all, it has pointed to the need to identify the political processes and lessons that can start to make a difference, and particularly the ways in which local and national action can be better integrated.

## References

Acheson, D. (1998) *Independent inquiry into inequalities in health*, London: The Stationery Office.

Ambrose, P. (2001) *A drop in the ocean: The health gain from the Central Stepney SRB in the context of national health inequalities*, Brighton: Health and Social Policy Research Centre, University of Brighton.

Archer, M. and Tritter, J.Q. (eds) (2000) *Rational choice theory: Resisting colonisation*, London and New York, NY: Routledge.

Arnott, D. and Willmore, I. (2006) 'Smoke and mirrors', *The Guardian*, 19 July.

Barnes, M., Bauld, L., Benzeval, M., McKenzie, M. and Sullivan, H. (2005) *Health Action Zones: Partnerships for health equity*, London: Routledge.

Bhaskar, R. (1978) *The possibility of naturalism*, Brighton: Harvester.

Blair, T. (2002) 'I have learned the limits of government', *Renewal: A Journal of Labour politics*, vol 10, no 2, pp 9–14.

Cabinet Office (2001) *A new commitment to neighbourhood renewal: national strategy action plan*, London: Social Exclusion Unit.

Carlisle, S. (2001) 'Inequalities in health: contested explanations, shifting discourses and ambiguous policies', *Critical Public Health*, vol 11, no 3, pp 267–81.

CDX (Community Development Exchange) (2006) *What is community development?*, Sheffield: Community Development Exchange (www.cdx.org.uk/about/whatiscd.htm).

Clark, T. (2003) 'Jam today', *The Guardian*, 30 January.

Coote, A., Allen, J. and Woodhead, D. (2004) *Finding out what works: Building knowledge about complex, community-based initiatives*, London: Kings Fund.

Craig, G. (1989) 'Community work and the state', *Community Development Journal*, vol 24, no 1, pp 3–18.

Curtis, S., Cave, B., and Coutts, A. (2002) *Regeneration and neighbourhood change*, London: Queen Mary, University of London (www.nice.org. uk/download.aspx?o=508193).

DH (2004) *Choosing health: Making healthier choices easier*, Cm 6374, London: The Stationery Office.

Doyal, L. and Gough, I. (1991) *A theory of human need*, Basingstoke: Macmillan.

Driver, S. and Martell, L. (2000) 'Left, right and the third way', *Policy and Politics*, vol 28, no 2, pp 147-61.

Exworthy, M., Bindman, A., Davies, H. and Washington, A.E. (2006) 'Evidence into policy and practice? Measuring the progress of U.S. and U.K. policies to tackle disparities and inequalities in U.S. and U.K. health and health care', *The Milbank Quarterly*, vol 84, no 1, pp 75-109.

Flank, F. and Smith, A. (1999) *The community development handbook: A tool to build community capacity*, Hull, Quebec: Human Resources Development Canada (www.hrsdc.gc.ca/en/gateways/topics/cyd-gxr.shtml).

Freire, P. (1986) *The pedagogy of the oppressed*, New York, NY: Continuum.

Fremeaux, I. (2005) 'New Labour's appropriation of the concept of community: a critique', *Community Development Journal*, vol 40, no 3, pp 265-74.

Gilchrist, A. (2003) 'Community development and networking for health', in J. Orme, J. Powell, P. Taylor, J. Harrison and M. Grey (eds) *Public health in the 21st century: New perspectives on policy, participation and practice*, Maidenhead: Open University Press, pp 145-60.

HDA (Health Development Agency) (2004a) *Lessons from Health Action Zones*, HDA Briefing No 9, London: HDA.

HDA (2004b) *Local government scrutiny and health*, HDA Briefing No 9, London: HDA.

HDA (2005) *Making the case: Health equity audit*, HDA Briefing, London: HDA.

Hills, D. (2004) *Evaluation of community-level interventions for health improvement: A review of experience in the UK*, London: Health Development Agency.

HM Treasury and DH (2002) *Tacking health inequalities: Summary of the 2002 cross-cutting review*, London: DH.

Judge, K. and Bauld, L. (2006) 'Learning from policy failure? Health Action Zones in England', *European Journal of Public Health*, vol 16, no 4, pp 341-3.

Kagan, C. (2006) 'Health hazards', *New Start*, vol 8, 13 January, pp 14-15.

Kawachi, I., Kim, D., Coutts, A. and Subramanian, S.V. (2004) 'Commentary: reconciling the 3 accounts of social capital', *International Journal of Epidemiology*, vol 33, no 4, pp 682-90.

Law, A. and Mooney, G. (2006) 'Social capital and neo-liberal voluntarism', *Variant*, no 26, pp 18-20 (www.variant.randomstate. org).

Ledwith, M. (2005) *Community development: A critical approach*, Bristol: The Policy Press.

Levitas, R. (1998) *The inclusive society: Social exclusion and New Labour*, Basingstoke: Macmillan.

Lynch, J.W., Davey Smith, G., Kaplan, G.A. and House, J.S. (2000) 'Income inequality and mortality: importance to health of individual income, psychosocial environment, or material conditions', *BMJ*, vol 320, 1200-4.

Moore, S., Haines, V., Hawe, P. and Shiell, A. (2006) 'Lost in translation: a genealogy of the "social capital" concept in public health', *Journal of Epidemiology and Community Health*, vol 60, no 8, pp 729-34.

Municipal Journal (2005) *Health inequalities: Rising to the challenge*, London: Health Inequalities Unit, Department of Health (www. dh.gov.uk/PolicyAndGuidance/HealthAndSocialCareTopics/ HealthInequalities/fs/en).

Nolan, P. (2004) 'The changing world of work', *Journal of Health Services Research and Policy*, vol 9, Supplement 1, no 1, pp 3-9.

Nutbeam, D. (1998) ' Evaluating health promotion – progress, problems and solutions', *Health Promotion International*, vol 13, no 1, pp 27-44.

ODPM (Office of the Deputy Prime Minister) (2005) *Creating healthier communities: A resource pack for local partnerships*, London: ODPM.

Pawson, R. and Tilley, N. (1997) *Realistic evaluation*, London: Sage Publications.

Putnam, R. (2000) *Bowling alone: The collapse and revival of American community*, New York, NY: Simon & Schuster.

Sassi, F. (2005) 'Tackling health inequalities' in J. Hills and K. Stewart (eds) *A more equal society? New Labour, poverty, inequality and exclusion*, Bristol: The Policy Press, pp 69-91.

Smithies, and Webster (1998) *Community involvement in health: From passive recipients to active participants*, Aldershot: Ashgate.

Szreter, S. and Woolcock, M. (2004) 'Health by association: social capital, social theory and the political economy of public health', reconciling the 3 accounts of social capital', *International Journal of Epidemiology*, vol 33, no 4, pp 650-67.

Taylor, M. (2003) *Public policy in the community*, Basingstoke: Palgrave Macmillan.

Thomson, H., Atkinson, R., Petticrew, M. and Kearns, A. (2006) 'Do urban regeneration programmes improve public health and reduce health inequalities? A synthesis of the evidence from UK policy and practice (1980-2004)', *Journal of Epidemiology and Community Health*, vol 60, no 2, pp 108-15.

Townsend, P., Davidson, N. and Whitehead, M. (1992) *The Black Report: The health divide*, Harmondsworth: Penguin.

UKPHA (United Kingdom Public Health Association) (2006) 'Natural and Built Environmental Strategic Interest Group', *Report: Newsletter of the UKPHA*, issue 20 (www.ukphaconference.org.uk/ukpha-newsletter-june.html).

WHO (World Health Organization) (1981) *Global strategy for health for all by the year 2000*, Geneva: WHO.

WHO (1986) *Ottawa Charter for health promotion*, Geneva: WHO (www.who.int/hpr/NPH/docs/ottawa_charter_hp.pdf).

Wilkinson, R. (1996) *Unhealthy societies: The afflictions of inequality*, London: Routledge.

Wilkinson, R. and Marmot, M. (eds) (2003) *Social determinants of health: The solid facts*, Copenhagen: WHO Regional Office for Europe (www.who.dk/document/e81384.pdf).

# TWELVE

# A new agenda for social work: tackling inequalities in physical health

*Eileen McLeod, Paul Bywaters, Peter Beresford, Suzy Croft and Mark Drakeford*

## Introduction

Unlike other disciplines represented in this book, a focus on addressing inequalities in physical health was not already established in social work discourse at the time of the Acheson Inquiry. However, in the intervening period, a major theoretical shift has occurred. Social work's contribution to tackling inequalities in physical health has gained recognition as a crucial component of theorising social work's engagement with inequality (Mullender, 1999; McLeod and Bywaters, 2000; Davies, 2002). The fundamental reasons why inequalities in physical health should be on social work's agenda are that:

- inequalities in physical health are endemic among social work service users;
- social work may compound social disadvantage implicated in unequal chances and experience of physical health;
- evidence is accumulating that social work generally – not simply in healthcare settings – that targets health inequalities and addresses unequal social conditions can contribute to more equal chances and experience of physical health.

In presenting this account, we are not perpetuating a false division between mental and physical health – our position is that physical and psychological well-being are intertwined – but registering the emergence of a further critical dimension to social work analysis. For the sake of brevity, in the remainder of the discussion physical health will be referred to as health.

## A pervasive problem

Social work service users are overwhelmingly drawn from people experiencing social disadvantage. Therefore it is not surprising that inequalities in health are endemic among them. The majority live in relative poverty (Jones, 2002), cross-cut by other dimensions to social disadvantage such as racism (Cambridge and Williams, 2004) and disability (Swain et al, 2003). Disproportionately high levels of ill health and inferior treatment in the course of ill health have, for example, been evidenced for care leavers (Broad, 2005), asylum seekers and refugees (Gray, 2003), and service users with learning disabilities or who are mental health service users (Kmietowicz, 2005). This should constitute a key issue for social work practice, as a situation of social injustice endured in individual pain and suffering (McLeod and Bywaters, 2002).

## Social work's complicity

Despite the prevalence of inferior health and healthcare among service users, social work's engagement with socially constructed health inequalities remains marginalised in social work policy and practice. Despite the then recently elected Labour government giving joint lead responsibility for tackling health inequalities to social services departments in England and Wales and the NHS (DH, 1998), there has remained little evidence of a systematic local authority social work response to this issue. This allocation of responsibility for health inequalities was overtaken by a concern to focus social services' role in relation to the NHS on alleviating pressures on acute hospital beds (McLeod et al, 2003). More recently the break-up of social services departments in English local authorities in favour of a division between children's and adult services has focused attention, once again, on organisational changes rather than the substance of policy (2004 Children Act; DH, 2005). It remains to be seen whether this corporate approach leads either to closer strategic links with the NHS through Primary Care Trusts (PCTs), to the addressing of inequalities in access to services, or to a better integration between social care and other local authority policies in addressing fundamental social and economic inequalities (Mahony, 2006).

When the public health White Paper, *Choosing health* (DH, 2004a), is considered, social services feature only as partners in local action on programmes such as the Teenage Pregnancy Partnership boards and the Communities for Health pilots, while in terms of their responsibility for looked after children, lead status clearly rests with PCTs. While the emphasis on individual decision making and professionals' guidance might seem to reinforce the potential role of social workers alongside health workers, the emphasis on fostering individual choice seems unlikely to reduce existing health inequalities (see Blaxter, 1990). The *Every child matters* framework (HM Government, 2004) places a clear requirement for social care services to encourage children to 'Be Healthy', but in doing so focuses on a series of individual behavioural measures (see Chapter Five of this volume for further discussion of the role of *Every child matters* in relation to health inequalities in the early years).

Moreover, resulting from persistent under-funding (Carvel, 2005) and ever narrower targeting of interventions, there is continued evidence of day-to-day social work practice failing to put in place adequate services. Such services providing enhanced resources in cash or kind would alleviate to some degree the material deprivation and complex social consequences that prejudice health and well-being across the life course (Lynch et al, 2000). The following two examples illustrate the significance of this diminution of services. Despite the attested benefits for health of preventive work (Clark et al, 1998), local social services teams have increasingly withdrawn from such service provision. While total contact hours have increased by 20%, the number of older people receiving home care through social services in England and Wales has reduced by 25% since 1996, despite the continuing rise in the population of older people (DH, 2004b). Even if local authority social workers may now be prohibited from carrying out detailed welfare rights work, ensuring that service users are advised on how to obtain financial benefits that are due to them does remain part of their brief. However, a report by Macmillan Cancer Relief in 2004 (Tunnage et al, 2004) found that despite social workers' involvement in home care and hospital care, about half the people who had died from cancer in 2001 had not claimed attendance allowance or disability living allowance.

## Social work tackling health inequalities

As we discuss in greater detail elsewhere (Bywaters and McLeod, 2001), enhanced funding for social work services, embedded in more thoroughgoing redistributive policies, is essential if social work's contribution to tackling inequalities in health is to be fully realised. Nevertheless, in an incremental way, new initiatives in social work practice are emerging that clearly bear on health inequalities. These developments are characterised by certain hallmarks. First, issues that have lain on the margins of mainstream practice have been reconfigured as a key focus for social work, in the interests of promoting greater equity in health and well-being. Safe housing provision, of a standard commensurate with health, is a case in point, as in projects concerning domestic violence (Humphreys et al, 2001), care leavers making the transition to independence (Broad, 2004) and support for teenage parents (Winchester, 2001; Tickle, 2004). Second, the prime movers in implementing such initiatives are not confined to the ranks of professional practitioners. Service users have gained recognition as strategists, practitioners and researchers (McLeod and Bywaters, 2000). Third, some of the most progressive examples of leverage on inequalities in physical health have come from the voluntary sector or activists previously unaligned to social work agencies, as in information activism, which has begun to identify and counter homophobic threats to health (see Mason and Palmer, 1996; Keogh et al, 2004). Finally, where social work is starting to deliver on health inequalities, it has also revised its repertoire of practice. It has, for example, reincorporated community action and contributed to the development of national networks, as in the campaign against the implementation of Do Not Resuscitate orders on ageist grounds, spearheaded by Age Concern (see Age Concern, 2000; Mayor, 2001).

These hallmarks of social work contributing to tackling health inequalities are illustrated in detail by the following two examples of practice. The first highlights the strategic importance of social work's role within community development anti-poverty initiatives, underwritten by Welsh Assembly health inequalities funding. Of course, Wales is not alone among the four UK nations in developing anti-poverty strategies drawing on skills germane to social work (see Waddington, 2004; Popple, 2006). However, our example illustrates both the importance of government policy – in this case through the Welsh Assembly – specifically supporting social work's engagement with health inequalities and the significance of that support being translated into the fine print of practice on a one-to-one, locality basis. The second example underlines the critical importance of user involvement in securing shifts in unequal professional–service user power relations. This is to increase the chances of healthcare promoting as opposed to disadvantaging service users' well-being. It analyses two initiatives that have increased patient/user representation in palliative care. It examines the first research project to obtain service users' feedback on specialist palliative care social work, and the significance of service user involvement in research governance. It then analyses the significance of the beginnings of palliative care service users' collective representation in the organisation and delivery of specialist palliative care services.

## Anti-poverty strategies in Wales

The relationship between health inequalities and social work is one that has been revived and reinforced by devolution in Wales. Since 1999, the Welsh Assembly has embarked on a distinctive social policy agenda (Chaney and Drakeford, 2004), most often summarised in the phrase coined by First Minister Rhodri Morgan when he spoke of the 'clear red water' that separated the policies being developed in Wales from those preferred in other parts of the United Kingdom (Morgan, 2002).

Among the principles that are claimed to be characteristic of this approach is a focus on creating a more equal society in Wales – not simply the pursuit of equality of opportunity, but as Morgan highlighted, the more fundamentally socialist objective of equality of outcome (Morgan, 2002). Health inequalities are amongst the most striking that face any administration attempting to pursue such an agenda. This chapter cannot hope to set out the facts that lie behind this claim in any detail (but see Greer, 2003a, 2003b; Sullivan and Drakeford, 2004). Suffice it to say that analysis of the 2001 census returns illustrates both the gap that separates those areas of Wales with best and worst health, and demonstrates, once again, the concentration of poorest health in the valley communities of South Wales (Doran et al, 2004; National Assembly for Wales, 2004).

Against this background, the Assembly invited Professor Peter Townsend to lead a project designed to produce a better match between the health needs of the Welsh population and the distribution of resources. The Townsend Report (2001) reached two major conclusions. It set out proposals to rectify a mismatch between the way in which health service money was allocated to different parts of Wales and the pattern of need on the ground. It also overlaid that allocative analysis with an insistence that health inequality could only be halted and reversed if the responsibility for doing so was shared among those services capable of influencing the determinants of health – economic development, housing, transport, environment and so on – rather than being laid at the NHS door alone.

Here, three initiatives are briefly discussed, each of which has been undertaken against the background of this 'dual strategy'. In each case, the argument presented will suggest that the contribution of social work approaches and principles are central to the success of what is being attempted.

## Reaching out

The widest of the three initiatives is the Health Inequalities Fund, a £14 million programme that, to date, has generated some 70 different projects in all parts of the country. Examples of practical action include healthy eating projects, mobile screening services and projects aimed at particular groups, such as pregnant teenagers and travellers. The fund is predicated on reaching out to those communities that are hardest to reach (see Chapter Ten for a detailed discussion of the concept of 'hard to reach') and where, in close conformity to the Tudor Hart inverse care law, services have often been weakest (National Assembly for Wales, 2004). In the case of the traveller project, for example, the scheme, based in Wrexham and known as Redressing the Balance, aims to improve access to healthcare services and to reduce and prevent the incidence of heart disease. Through a full-time project worker and purchase of a specially equipped mobile unit, it has enabled 200 Gypsy Travellers to be offered health screening, advice and support, which is both accessible and acceptable. Over 95% of the community are now registered with a general practitioner (family doctor). By providing an on-site service, it has identified those most at risk of coronary heart disease, through monitoring blood pressure and addressing issues such as high cholesterol, exercise, obesity, nutrition and smoking (personal communication, ministerial briefing, 2004).

Interim evaluation of all of the fund's projects has been reported to the Assembly Health and Social Services Committee (Welsh Assembly Government, 2002). Second-stage evaluation is in progress and draft available evidence suggests (personal communication, 2006) that where successful, the fund's approach has relied on close attention to community needs, willingness to listen and learn as well as to preach and teach, and multidisciplinary teamwork that overcomes traditional professional demarcations. In some projects, local authority social workers are directly involved in service provision. In others, the cadre of new welfare workers – variously described as community workers, project workers and so on – share a trait that Jordan (2001; 2004) has identified as characteristic of the post-1997 era, an eager willingness to embrace ways of working that have been the province of social work, while fighting shy of employing the term itself.

## Better benefits access

Better Advice, Better Health works as a partnership between the National Association of Citizens Advice Bureaux (CABs) in Wales and the Welsh Assembly, which provides annual funding to the tune of £700,000. That sum secures the provision of a service in all 22 local health board areas in Wales, in which welfare benefits advice is provided directly in primary care settings. The project was predicated on research that underscored two key conclusions. First, the failure to take up benefits is a particular problem among two groups that, at the same time, are major users of primary care services – the vulnerable elderly and people with chronic mental health problems – and second, the striking success with which barriers to take-up could be overcome if advice were provided directly in GP surgeries. The connection between poverty and chronic illness is one that needs no explanation for health workers in many parts of Wales, yet the take-up of the minimum income guarantee among vulnerable groups such as single women aged 75 was the worst of any group in the population (McConaghy et al, 2003). The evaluation report (Borland and Owens, 2004), completed after the initial round of funding, found that the programme had exceeded its targets in all dimensions – operating from more outlets than planned, seeing more people than predicted and raising more than £3.5 million in annual unclaimed benefits among the poorest. With £5 raised for every £1 invested, the Welsh Assembly Health Minister moved quickly to implement core long-term funding for the programme.

Once again, the connections between social work and the Better Advice, Better Health programme are clear. There is an obvious overlap between the client groups on whom the scheme concentrates and those who are users of social work services. The skills that advice workers require are those that social workers have routinely to employ – an ability to win the confidence of the wary; to explore, with a minimum of preamble, some very personal information that individuals may not otherwise share widely; to translate this information into practical action in which the worker acts as a broker between the user and a major service of the welfare state.

There is a long and honourable tradition in social work that emphasises the obligation to deal directly with the underlying causes of social distress, rather than the symptoms of family and individual difficulty such conditions create (Becker, 1997; Craig, 2002; Drakeford, 2002a). Better Advice, Better Health arises straight from that tradition. It looks to put money into the pockets of those who most need it, in the belief that this will have a direct impact on the conditions – cold, damp, under-nourishment – that produce chronic ill health. In doing so, it removes the cause, rather than simply ameliorates the symptoms, of the problem.

## Credit union services

The same focus on poverty, inequality and health is to be found in the third initiative reported here, drawn from the work of the credit union movement in Wales, a movement that, it has been argued (see Drakeford, 2002b) has developed in a way that is different from the rest of the UK. In both England and Scotland (Ryder, 2003), the drive to expand the coverage of credit unions has focused on the need to broaden the base of membership by shaking off their image as 'poor people's banks'. In Wales, the same determination to increase the reach of credit unions has focused on expanding their range of services, thus making them more attractive to potential members and especially those in the most disadvantaged circumstances. A number of examples of this diversification have focused on making fuel bills easier to manage, either by offering fuel-efficient goods – kettles, fridges – at very cheap rates to credit union members, or by entering into arrangements with fuel companies to make direct debit tariffs available through credit unions to individuals who might otherwise have to depend on far more expensive pre-payment meters.

For this chapter, however, it is worth highlighting an idea that operates even more directly in the health field. The problems that paying for prescriptions cause for individuals whose incomes lie just above income support levels have been well documented (NACAB, 1999; Galvin et al, 2000; Emanuel, 2002). For people with chronic diseases, in particular, multiple prescriptions may be needed to keep conditions properly under control. The NHS provides a 'season ticket' system in which a single payment can cover all prescriptions needed over a four- or twelve-month period. The problem for those who need this facility the most is, of course, that they are least able to afford the down payment required of a pre-payment certificate (as it is known).

Normal credit union operation cannot cater for such a difficulty, because a loan to cover such a lump-sum payment depends on having run up a savings record with the union of at least eight consecutive weeks in advance of any loan being made. Now, through an arrangement with the Welsh Assembly, some credit unions in Wales can make the lump sum available to patients immediately the need arises. Referrals to the scheme can be made through the Better Health, Better Advice projects discussed above. On being given a loan, individuals become members of their local credit union in the normal way, repaying the amount advanced and building up a savings record. Clearly, there are risks involved for unions in lending money to people of whom they have no previous knowledge. The Welsh Assembly acts as a guarantor against loss, unlocking the potential for a benign circle to be created in which credit unions gain new members, those new members are provided with an immediate financial benefit and the risk is removed that, otherwise, choices would have to be made between different forms of medication on the basis of affordability rather than health need.[1]

The principles on which credit unions operate – mutuality, equality, harnessing collective strength to promote individual improvement – are an exact fit with the sort of social work this chapter has sought to advance, one that is directly and positively engaged with the needs of its users and determined to address the underlying causes of difficulty rather than simply relieving its symptoms.

## Specialist palliative care social work and user involvement: two case studies

Our second example of the possibilities and problems of social work contributing to tackling inequalities in health is centred on promoting service user involvement in specialist palliative care social work (SPCSW). It draws on two case studies: the first a research initiative, the second concerning user involvement in the organisation of palliative care.

Practitioners in this branch of social work primarily work in multidisciplinary teams integral to hospice care. The hospice movement, operating in the voluntary sector, engages with two groups of service users: people with life-limiting illnesses and people facing and experiencing bereavement. Its fundamental commitment is to a holistic approach to health/social care, which seeks to address people's physical, emotional, cultural and spiritual selves in their broader social and political context. (Oliviere et al, 1998). Through the services it provides, it also seeks to facilitate people's choice of where they die. Currently, much more support tends to be provided on a 'hospice at home' basis to people where they live than on an in-hospice basis. Accordingly, a large part of SPCSW social workers' time is spent with people in their own homes (Croft et al, 2005).

While social work generally tends to have low status and a poor press, this does not seem to be true of SPCSW. In public debate, it has been positively associated with a highly valued area of health and welfare provision – hospice and palliative care services (Monroe and

Oliviere, 2003); however, ironically, SPCSW tends to be marginalised in mainstream social work discourse, compared, for example, with child protection and work with families and young people (McLeod and Bywaters, 2000). Moreover, systematic evidence on the nature and quality of SPCSW, based on feedback from service users, has not been available.

## User involvement: research

To address this dearth of evidence, the authors of this chapter recently completed a three-year project, supported by the Joseph Rowntree Foundation, that explored service users' views on the SPCSW service they received (Croft et al, 2005). It explored with service users the process and outcomes of practice and their ideas for improving provision. A total of 111 service users were interviewed nationally in the project: 61 bereaved people, and 52 people with life-limiting illnesses and conditions (two people were both bereaved and patients). It was a diverse sample, including Black and minority ethnic service users, people aged from 18 to 80, living with cancer and a range of other life-limiting conditions, from town, city and country and from a wide range of class and occupational backgrounds. They also came from a wide range of palliative care settings, including both statutory and voluntary services, day hospitals, hospices and palliative care units. In undertaking this work, it was evident that service users who *had* managed to access palliative care services tended to be in a relatively advantaged position, as access bears the imprint of social inequalities. Only a small proportion of the population with life-limiting illnesses and conditions accesses palliative care services, and an even smaller proportion accesses support from SPCSW (Gott et al, 2001). Black and minority ethnic service users have inferior access to specialist palliative care (Hill and Penso, 1995; Karim et al, 2000; Koffman and Higginson, 2001). There are also indications that access is class-based, with working-class patients having inferior access (Oliviere and Monroe, 2004). Other groups identified as significantly less likely to access SPCSW include mental health service users, people with learning difficulties, disabled people and older people (Croft, 1996).

Nevertheless, the study provided the opportunity for service users to begin to map, through systematic research, the features of SPCSW that they found contributed to their well-being, as opposed to the definition of such factors continuing to be bounded by professional assumptions – potentially to service users' detriment (Monroe and Oliviere, 2003). Here we highlight briefly two distinctive features of this work: first, how service users were assisted to undertake a lead role in the research and some indication of the difference this made to research design and the quality of material; and second, how palliative care social work might be developed in service users' interests.

From the outset, a participatory approach was employed in undertaking the research, to support active and effective service user involvement and to make participation in the project as positive an experience as possible. This included, for example, providing detailed accessible information to underwrite informed consent, providing a newsletter to keep research participants in touch with the project and offering follow-up support through a card maintaining personal contact, and encouraging people to speak to a specialist social worker if they wanted to. The project was overseen by an advisory group including specialist palliative care (and other) service users. It was also guided by a series of steering groups made up of palliative care service users, who commented on and influenced the design of the research interview schedule. These steering groups worked well. In some cases, they had a rotating membership as some service users died, as might be expected, during the course of the project. Involving service users in the management of the project helped both to focus it on issues of major concern to participants and to ensure that questions were clear and meaningful to them and sensitive to their often difficult circumstances.

Participants were almost universally positive about their experience of SPCSW practice, although as researchers we tried hard to enable them to highlight any negative aspects. They had found it helpful and supportive, improving their quality of life and capacity to cope with the major difficulties and changes they had been experiencing. Service users particularly commented on valuing the quality of the relationship with the social worker. They appreciated its flexibility and the range of support provided. This seemed to have been skilfully tailored to meet individual service users' different needs and preferences.

A minority of service users did identify some shortcomings in SPCSW, but these related much more to its *management* than to the quality of direct practice. Some service users, for example, wished that SPCSW had been made available to them earlier on in their contact with palliative care services, when they were already encountering serious emotional, social and financial problems associated with life-limiting illness. However, referral by palliative healthcare staff still seemed to be influenced by a medical model, that is, one based on service users' severity of physical symptoms, rather than the extent of their emotional and practical difficulties. Thus patients were predominantly referred to social work for medical reasons, although many stressed how important the social worker had been in supporting them in their psychological difficulties.

Service users also recommended that healthcare professionals generally should adopt a more systematic approach to referral, through routinely informing potential service users about SPCSW and enabling them to access social work support. Extensive practice experience also endorsed the need for a more systematic approach. It suggested that medical professionals – within and outside palliative care – tend to refer on the basis of stereotypes of who would benefit and, no less worryingly, preconceptions of SPCSW (for example, associating such social work with 'devalued' people).

The study also indicated that a disproportionately small number of men and Black and minority ethnic service users seemed to be referred (Croft et al, 2005). In service users' interests, these aspects of the management of referral constitute important issues for further research and practice to address.

## User involvement: policy

Our second case study provides an example of how collective user involvement can be promoted in the organisation of palliative care. It illustrates how user involvement – on which the government now places such emphasis generally, and specifically in relation to health and social care (DH, 2003) – can begin to exert leverage on the quality of services and support people receive (see Chapter Ten for a detailed discussion of the role of user involvement in challenging health inequalities). It also challenges disablist assumptions that SPCSW service users per se are unable to undertake such initiatives because of the life-limiting nature of their illness (McLeod and Bywaters, 2000).

Social work and social care have been important sites for pioneering and developing effective policy and practice for user involvement (Beresford and Croft, 1993; Carr, 2004; Beresford et al, 2005). Briefly, what we have learned from these developments is that user involvement to improve services is both feasible and valuable, for example, through:

- systematic user involvement in training and education – a key route to culture change (Levin, 2004);
- user involvement in monitoring and evaluation, to include service users' perspectives and interpretations (Evans, 1996);
- developing user-defined outcome measures and other standards

that identify what service users want, value and prioritise, rather than just reinforcing the service system's concerns or the targets it is required to meet (Beresford et al, 2000);

* enabling *diverse* involvement that addresses difference and social divisions, particularly concerning issues of gender, age, sexuality, culture, disability and race equality (Beresford and Croft, 1993; Morris, 1996; Oliviere and Monroe, 2004).

What is particularly interesting about palliative care and SPCSW is that they have frequently been seen as areas where such user involvement might not be possible, either for *practical* reasons – how could you effectively involve service users who were very ill, would probably die soon, would be likely to have little time and other pressing priorities? – or for *ethical* reasons – how could you justify *ethically* involving such people at such difficult times in their lives (Small and Rhodes, 2000)?

Through our working experience and research, both objections can be properly met (Oliviere, 2000; Beresford et al, 2001; Kraus et al, 2003). People who are very ill can and want to be involved and it is possible to involve them on both an individual and group basis. It requires imagination, sensitivity and support.

Service users often express a desire to make such a contribution to help others who turn to the same services. As one young woman who participated in our research project said to us:

> "I am quite happy to do this because I feel as though I am giving something back ... perhaps people who come along afterwards [can] benefit from that, you know, from other people's experience." (Croft et al, 2005, p 20)

There are real gains for policy and practice from such involvement. Palliative care service users, like other service users, have important experiential knowledge to contribute to the evidence base for policy and services.

We have been involved in a number of joint initiatives with palliative care service users, some of whom were also users of SPCSW. In this way, palliative care service users have been involved for the first time in the UK in planning – as equal partners with professional representatives – a national conference and seminar as well as regional seminars, in judging palliative care awards and in developing ongoing user involvement in national policy organisations, including Help the Hospices and the National Council for Palliative Care (Beresford et al, 2000). Our own contacts with initiatives across the UK indicate that this is now leading to palliative care service users beginning to be involved at local, regional and national levels: in local audit and local user groups, in quality assessment, and in the National Cancer Research Network. By drawing on knowledge that comes from people's own direct experience, as a key source of evidence, these initiatives have a crucial role in ensuring that the process of developing policy, practice, management, services and support is exposed to service users' requirements. By developing imaginative outreach approaches, it is also possible to ensure a level of diversity in service users' involvement that can help identify and challenge forms of exclusion and discrimination. This is already beginning to happen with, for example, the establishment of IT-based 'virtual' user groups with people with motor neurone disease, as a means of enabling wider service user involvement in advising research projects; and in the growth of work specifically with people with learning difficulties facing life-limiting illnesses and conditions, and bereavement.

As these two case studies from SPCSW illustrate, inequality in the provision of health and social care services takes diverse forms. These include professional–service user hierarchies, inequality of access and unequal experiences of the process of service provision. Social work and social care have pioneered and developed ideas of 'anti-discriminatory' and 'anti-oppressive' practice. Such principles, combined with the development of collective user involvement, not only provide a basis for more comprehensive understandings of inequalities in health/social care provision but also for more effective responses.

## Conclusion

This chapter has shown how, since the time of the Acheson Inquiry, incremental improvements in unequal health chances and experience have resulted from the issue of tackling health inequalities coming on to the social work agenda. Nevertheless, this account has also underscored how social work remains constrained by the tenor of policies and social relations more generally. Further, it has pointed to the need for developments in policy, research and practice specifically related to social work, to optimise its contribution to addressing inequalities in health. Inescapably, these include measures to address perennial under-funding (Wanless, 2006). Social work's policy briefs – from central government to team level – need to identify the promotion of more equal chances of physical and psychological health as a core objective. Research is required that both traces the impact of initiatives with such goals and places service users at the forefront of research design, delivery and dissemination. Finally, as an interactive, interventive discipline, social work is nothing without its practice. The detailed examples discussed here illustrate the possibility and importance of refashioning and developing social work's modes of operating: to engage with service users' daily experience of health inequalities, to target underlying social inequalities, and to build collective service user strength in the interests of their health.

## Note

[1] Since this chapter was written, prescription charges have been abolished in Wales.

## References

Age Concern (2000) *Information on resuscitation*, London: Age Concern England.

Becker, S. (1997) *Responding to poverty: The politics of cash and care*, London: Longman.

Beresford, P. and Croft, S. (1993) *Citizen involvement: A practical guide for change*, Basingstoke: Macmillan.

Beresford, P., Broughton, F., Croft, S., Fouquet, S., Oliviere, D. and Rhodes, P. (2000) *Improving quality, developing user involvement*, Middlesex: Centre for Citizen Participation, Brunel University.

Beresford, P., Croft, S., Adshead, L., Walker, J. and Wilman, K. (2005) 'Involving service users in palliative care: from theory to practice', in P. Firth, G. Luff, and D. Oliviere (eds) *Loss, change and bereavement in palliative care*, Maidenhead: Open University Press, pp 119-32.

Beresford, P., Croft, S. and Oliviere, D. (2001) *Our lives, not our illness: User involvement in palliative care*, Briefing Paper 6, London: National Council for Hospice and Specialist Palliative Care Services.

Blaxter, M. (1990) *Health and lifestyles*, London: Routledge.

Borland, J. and Owens, D. (2004) *Welfare advice in general practice – the Better Advice, Better Health project in Wales*, Cardiff: National Assembly for Wales.

Broad, B. (2004) 'Obstacles on the pathway', *Community Care*, 8 July, pp 32-3.

Broad, B. (2005) *Improving the health and well-being of young people leaving care*, Lyme Regis: Russell House Publishers.

Bywaters, P. and McLeod, E. (2001) 'The impact of New Labour health policy on social services: a New Deal for service users' health?', *British Journal of Social Work*, vol 31, no 4, pp 579-94.

Cambridge, P. and Williams, L. (2004) 'Approaches to advocacy for refugees and asylum seekers: a development case study for a local support and advice service', *Journal of Refugee Studies*, vol 17, no 1, pp 97–113.

Carr, S. (2004) *Has service user participation made a difference to social care services?*, Position Paper No 3, London: Social Care Institute for Excellence.

Carvel, J. (2005) 'Age shall not weary him', *The Guardian: Social Care Supplement*, 2 February, p 10.

Chaney, P. and Drakeford, M. (2004) 'The primacy of ideology: social policy and the first term of the National Assembly for Wales', in N. Ellison, L. Bauld and M. Powell (eds) *Social Policy Review 16*, Bristol: The Policy Press, pp 121–42.

Clark, H., Dyer, S. and Horwood, J. (1998) *That bit of help: The high value of low level preventative services for older people*, Bristol: The Policy Press and Joseph Rowntree Foundation.

Craig, G (2002) 'Poverty, social work and social justice', *British Journal of Social Work*, vol 32, no 6, pp 669–82.

Croft, S. (1996) 'How can I leave them?: towards an empowering social work practice with women who are dying', in B. Fawcett, M. Galloway, and J. Perrin (eds) *Feminism and social work in the year 2000: Conflicts and controversies, report of a national conference*, Bradford: University of Bradford, pp 74–89.

Croft, S., Adshead, L. and Beresford, P. (2005) *What service users want from specialist palliative care social work*, York: York Publishing Services.

Davies, M. (2002) 'Introduction', in M. Davies (ed) *The Blackwell companion to social work* (2nd edn), Oxford: Blackwell Publishers.

DH (Department of Health) (1998) *Modernising health and social services: National priorities guidance 1999/00–2001/02*, London: DH.

DH (2003) *Building on the best: Choice, responsiveness and equity in the NHS*, Cm 6079, London: DH.

DH (2004a) *Choosing health: Making healthier choices easier*, Cm 6374, London: The Stationery Office.

DH (2004b) *Health and personal social services statistics*, Table c6, London: DH (www.performance.doh.gov.uk/HPSSS/TBL_C6.HTM).

DH (2005) *Independence, well-being and choice. Our vision for the future of social care in England*, London: DH.

Doran, T., Drever, T. and Whitehead, M. (2004) 'Is there a north–south divide in social class inequalities in health in Great Britain? Cross sectional study using data from the 2001 census', *British Medical Journal*, vol 328, pp 1043–5.

Drakeford, M. (2002a) 'Poverty and the social services', in B. Bytheway, V. Bacigalupo, J. Bornat, J. Johnson and S. Spurr (eds), *Understanding care, welfare and community*, Buckingham: Open University Press.

Drakeford, M. (2002b) 'Co-ordinating policies and powers to reduce social exclusion: the Welsh approach to credit union development', *Welsh Journal of Law and Policy*, vol 1, p 3.

Emanuel, J. (2002) 'Citizens Advice Bureaux in primary care: a tool to address social and economic inequalities', in L. Adams, M. Amos and J. Munro (eds) *Promoting health policy and practice*, London: Sage Publications.

Evans, C. (1996) 'Service users acting as agents of change', in P. Bywaters and E. McLeod (eds) *Working for equality in health*, London: Routledge, pp 81-93.

Galvin, K., Sharples, A. and Jackson, D. (2000) 'Citizens Advice Bureaux in general practice: an illuminative evaluation', *Health and Social Care in the Community*, vol 8, no 4, pp 277-82.

Gott, C.M., Ahmedzai, S.H., and Wood, C. (2001) 'How many inpatients at an acute hospital have palliative care need? Comparing the perspectives of medical and nursing staff', *Palliative Medicine*, vol 15, no 6, pp 451-60.

Gray, B. (2003) 'Social exclusion, poverty, health and social care in Tower Hamlets: the perspectives of families on the impact of the family support service', *British Journal of Social Work*, vol 33, no 3, pp 361-80.

Greer, S. (2003a) 'Health: how far can Wales diverge from England?', in J. Osmond (ed) *Second term challenge: Can the Welsh Assembly Government hold its course?*, Cardiff: Institute of Welsh Affairs, pp 89-118.

Greer, S. (2003b) 'Policy divergence', in R. Hazell (ed) *The state of the nation 2003: The third year of devolution in the United Kingdom*, Exeter: Imprint Academic, pp 54-72.

Hill, D. and Penso, D. (1995) *Opening doors: Improving access to hospice and specialist care services by members of black and ethnic minority communities*, Occasional Paper 7, London: National Council for Hospice and Specialist Palliative Care Services.

HM Government (2004) *Every child matters: Change for children*, London: HMSO.

Humphreys, C., Mullender, A., Lowe, P., Hague, G., Abrahams, H. and Hester, M. (2001) 'Domestic violence and child abuse: developing sensitive policies and guidance', *Child Abuse Review*, vol 10, no 3, pp 183-97.

Jones, C. (2002) 'Poverty and social exclusion', in M. Davies (ed) *The Blackwell companion to social work* (2nd edn), Oxford: Blackwell Publishers.

Jordan, B. (2001) 'Tough love: social work, social exclusion and the Third Way', *British Journal of Social Work*, vol 3, no 4, pp 527-46.

Jordan, B. (2004) 'The personal social services', in N. Ellison, L. Bauld and M. Powell (eds) *Social Policy Review 16*, Bristol: The Policy Press, pp 81-98.

Karim, K., Bailey, M. and Tunna, K. (2000) 'Non white ethnicity and the provision of specialist palliative care services: factors affecting doctors' referral patterns', *Palliative Medicine*, vol 14, no 6, pp 471-8.

Keogh, P., Weatherburn, P., Henderson, L., Reid, D., Dodds, C. and Hickson, F. (2004) *Doctoring gay men: Exploring the contribution of General Practice*, London: Sigma Research (www.sigmaresearch.org. uk/reports).

Kmietowicz, Z. (2005) 'Poorer health among disabled people to be investigated', *British Medical Journal*, vol 330, pp 8-9.

Koffman, J. and Higginson, I. (2001) 'Accounts of carers' satisfaction with health care at the end of life: a comparison of first generation black Caribbeans and white patients with advanced disease', *Palliative Medicine*, vol 15, no 4, pp 337-45.

Kraus, F., Levy, J. and Oliviere, D. (2003) 'Brief report on user involvement at St Christopher's Hospice', *Palliative Medicine*, vol 17, no 6, pp 375-7.

Levin, E. (2004) *Involving service users and carers in social work education*, Resource Guide No 2, London: Social Care Institute for Excellence.

Lynch, J., Davey Smith, G., Kaplan, G. and House, J. (2000) 'Income inequality and mortality: importance to health of individual income, psychosocial environment or material conditions', *British Medical Journal*, vol 320, pp 1200-4.

Mahony, C. (2006) 'A golden thread, but some hands are still tied', *The Guardian, Society Guardian*, 14 June.

Mason, A. and Palmer, A. (1996) *Queerbashing: A national survey of hate crimes against lesbians and gay men*, London: Stonewall.

Mayor, S. (2001) 'New UK guidance on resuscitation calls for open decision making', *British Medical Journal*, vol 322, p 509.

McConaghy, M., Hill, C., Kane, C., Laader, D., Constigan, P. and Thornby, M. (2003) *Entitled but not claiming? Pensioners, the minimum income guarantee and pension credit*, London: Office for National Statistics.

McLeod, E. and Bywaters, P. (2000) *Social work, health and equality*, London: Routledge.

McLeod, E. and Bywaters, P. (2002) 'Ill-health', in M. Davies (ed) *The Blackwell companion to social work* (2nd edn), Oxford: Blackwell Publishers.

McLeod, E., Bywaters, P. and Cooke, M. (2003) 'Social work in accident and emergency departments: a better deal for older patients' health?', *British Journal of Social Work*, vol 33, no 6, pp 787–802.

Monroe, B. and Oliviere, D. (2003) *Patient participation in palliative care: A voice for the voiceless*, Oxford: Oxford University Press.

Morgan, R. (2002) 'Making social policy in Wales', Lecture by the First Minister Rhodri Morgan to the Centre for Policy Studies, Swansea.

Morris, J. (ed) (1996) *Encounters with strangers: Feminism and disability*, London: Women's Press.

Mullender, A. (1999) 'Editorial', *British Journal of Social Work*, vol 29, no 4, pp 509–11.

NACAB (National Association of Citizens Advice Bureaux) (1999) *Prescribing advice*, London: NACAB.

National Assembly for Wales (2004) *Welsh Health Survey: October 2003–March 2004 (provisional results)*, SDR 82/2004, Cardiff: National Statistical Directorate.

Oliviere, D. (2000) 'A voice for the voiceless', *European Journal of Palliative Care*, vol 7, no 3, pp 102–5.

Oliviere, D. and Monroe, B. (eds) (2004) *Death, dying and social differences*, Oxford: Oxford University Press.

Oliviere, D., Hargreaves, R. and Monroe, B. (1998) *Good practices in palliative care*, Aldershot: Ashgate Arena.

Popple, K. (2006) 'Critical commentary: community development in the 21st century: a case of conditional development', *British Journal of Social Work*, vol 36, no 2, pp 333–40.

Ryder, N. (2003) 'Credit union development in Wales – an extension of the Westminster model?', *Welsh Journal of Law and Policy*, vol 2, p 4.

Small, N. and Rhodes, P. (2000) *Too ill to talk? User involvement and palliative care*, London: Routledge.

Sullivan, M. and Drakeford, M. (2004) 'Devolution, divergence and social policy', *Welsh Journal of Law and Policy*, vol 2, p 4.

Swain, J., French, S. and Cameron, C. (2003) *Controversial issues in a disabling society,* Maidenhead: Open University Press.

Tickle, L. (2004) 'Building support', *Community Care*, 1 July, pp 32–3.

Townsend, P. (2001) *Targeting poor health*, Cardiff: Welsh Assembly Government.

Tunnage, B., Tudor Edwards, R. and Linck, P. (2004) *Estimation of the extent of unclaimed Disability Living Allowance and Attendance Allowance for people with a terminal diagnosis of cancer*, Bangor: Centre for the Economics of Health, University of Wales, Bangor.

Waddington, D. (2004) '"Making the difference" in Warsop Vale: the impact of government regeneration policy and community development on a Nottinghamshire ex-mining community', *Social Policy and Society*, vol 3, no 1, pp 21-31.

Wanless, D. (2006) *Securing good care for older people: Taking a long-term view*, London: King's Fund.

Welsh Assembly Government (2002) *The Inequalities in Health Fund: An interim evaluation report to the Health and Social Services Committee (July)*, Cardiff: Welsh Assembly Government (www.cmo. wales.gov.uk/content/work/inequalities-in-health-fund/interim-evaluation-e.pdf).

Winchester, R. (2001) 'Housing's wider role', *Community Care*, 20 September, Supplement, pp iv-vi.

# THIRTEEN

# Challenging health inequalities: themes and issues

*Elizabeth Dowler and Nick Spencer*

This book engages with the contemporary challenge of health inequalities in rich, industrialised countries, with particular focus on the UK, drawing on different disciplinary perspectives and policy instruments. It reviews the trajectories of problem analysis and policy responses following the *Independent inquiry into inequalities in health* (Acheson, 1998) in England and Wales, which was set up and published early in the heady days of the New Labour government, elected in the UK with a landslide victory in 1997 on a mandate to reduce 'unacceptable inequalities in health' among other ills. Even at the time, the process of the inquiry, with its consultations, background briefing papers and choice of policy areas, seemed fresh, appropriate and full of exciting promise. Perhaps it was inevitable that there should be disappointment; the accounts given here, while sometimes reminiscent of the caricatured curate's response to his egg of merely 'good in parts', largely conclude that things could in fact have been better (cf Chapter Three).

There have clearly been some social policy achievements, such as the reductions in child poverty (see Chapter Five) and the introduction – and uprating – of a minimum wage. Stopping smoking is no longer entirely left to 'education versus the free market' (Chapter Nine), and another of the main determinants of health – diet – has risen up the policy agenda, such that the worst excesses of market liberalism in the food system are being acknowledged, with attention to school meals, food labelling and advertising (see Chapter Eight; Morgan, 2006). Also, reflecting contemporary notions of involvement and consultation, policies that try to engage with local people, whether characterised as residents, users or patients, have been initiated – and often rapidly changed – as discussed in Chapters Ten and Eleven. They too highlight some achievements, both in general and through specific examples of the involvement of people with serious mental health problems or who are homeless. These, among other examples of good practice documented throughout the volume, do point to serious attempts to understand causality upstream and downstream and to put appropriate instruments in place to address the challenges identified. In Chapter Two, Ray Earwicker gives a cogent account of the internal mechanisms of government necessary to achieve upstream change, although within the confines of a contributory chapter and his current position, he perhaps has limited space and personal agency to explore detailed reasons for policy shift.

That there has been a policy shift is a common thread throughout the book. Most authors in this volume, including Earwicker, lament the loss of an explicit inequalities focus in the late 2004 public health White Paper *Choosing health* (DH, 2004). In addition, Chapters Three, Four, Eight, Nine and Eleven all highlight an apparent major change of policy direction in this publication, from the materialist, structural approach adopted by the Acheson Inquiry (Acheson, 1998) and subsequent White Paper (DH, 1999), albeit in partnership with communities and people, back towards lifestyle and behaviourist approaches, with a focus on the individual's responsibilities that characterised policy under the pre-1997 administration. The introduction to the earlier White Paper *Saving lives: Our healthier nation* (DH, 1999) includes the statement: 'We believe that the social, economic and environmental factors tending towards poor health are potent' (DH, 1999, p ix). *Choosing health*, by contrast, sets out as its key principle 'informed choice': 'helping people to make healthier choices for themselves; protecting people's health from the actions of others' (DH, 2004, p 6). Its targets are nearly all behavioural and its means are supporting rational, informed individual choice of new ways of behaving (in relation to tobacco, diet, physical activity and so on). That this is justified by reference to extensive public consultation is neither here nor there (similar consultations preceded the 1999 public health White Paper); the policy shift is more a reflection of New Labour's current 'mantra of choice and individualism combined with market-style incentives to modify lifestyles' (Hunter, 2005, p 1010). In both White Papers, there is recognition of both people's and governmental responsibilities for bringing about better public health, but the ordering and significance has been reversed. In 1999, building on the Acheson Inquiry, the government both led and concentrated action on 'factors which harm people's health which are beyond the control of the individual' (DH, 1999, p ix). Government takes a relative back seat by 2004, a 'supporting' role, embracing social marketing and personalisation, and looking to develop partnerships with the many different actors – public and private sector – whose actions affect health outcomes.

Although many of the initiatives discussed earlier have the potential to reduce health inequalities, key fundamental drivers such as income distribution have worsened over the decade (see Chapters Three and Four). Current strategies seem more designed to 'raise the floor', to lift those on the lowest incomes, including those living on state benefits of various kinds, to something approaching a reasonable minimum for decent living, rather than addressing inequalities of wealth and opportunity across the whole range (Chapters Three and Eleven; Shaw et al, 2005). Whether inequalities in *health* can be fully addressed without redressing inequalities in *income*, and if so, how this might best be achieved, is currently much debated in academic and policy literatures (Emberson et al, 2004; Graham and Kelly, 2004; Marmot, 2004a; Judge et al, 2006; Lynch et al, 2006). Research is also emerging on the role of welfare regimes and practice (Adams et al, 2006; Dahl et al, 2006). The debate tends to be couched in terms of reducing the effects of social determinants – that is, controlling 'risk factors' – and whether efforts should focus on the worst off or the whole population. Most recognise that 'risk factors' are embedded in the social, political and cultural environments in which people live, and many use a life-course framework to highlight cumulative disadvantage (Chapters Four and Nine; Davey Smith, 2003; Asthana and Halliday, 2006). Indeed, as Marmot put it: 'We ... need to pay attention to the causes of inequalities in health, and the Acheson report suggested 39 ways that this could be done, starting from the beginnings of life and carrying through to old age. We also need to pay attention to risk factors' (Marmot, 2004a, p 298). However, Marmot, in common with many, goes on to call for building inequalities specifically into programmes and policies. Whether or not this has been successfully done in terms of targets or objectives over the past decade in the UK, and this too is debatable, the effects have been to widen inequalities in outcome.

The present government is driven by 'evidence-based policy', but establishing what kind of intervention to reduce inequalities gives the best return for investment is not a simple scientific calculation: valuing certain gains over others is as much a social and political decision. Chapters Eleven and Twelve discuss these issues and their implications, as do Chapters Six and Seven in terms of performance monitoring and regulatory challenges. Furthermore, as Asthana and Halliday (2006) comment, there is still very little evidence available on the effectiveness of interventions to address health inequalities, as opposed to health determinants in general, with the effects on socioeconomic groups as a category among many. This, as Asthana and Halliday (2006) point out, is in part because of the problematic hierarchy of evidence acceptability: few social or community/population-based initiatives lend themselves to systematic evaluative methods such as Randomised Controlled Trials (although there are exceptions – see Watts et al, 2006, and Thorogood et al, 2007, for examples of dietary intervention evaluations), so that effectiveness is difficult to demonstrate to the satisfaction of professionals responsible for advice, establishing or implementation of policy. In common with Asthana and Halliday (2006) and others, Mick Carpenter (Chapter Eleven) calls for a new 'mixed economy' framework for evidence-based public health, wherein social welfare initiatives that address inequalities can be more readily and appropriately assessed.

The chapters in this volume challenge health inequalities from different sectoral and disciplinary perspectives, but there are two important themes emerging from them that bear further examination in a concluding chapter. The first is the nature of the inequalities and how they are defined, including the relationships between health and income, social status, life chances, and the interplay between individual, household or neighbourhood experiences and effects. Second, in the fields represented here as in others, the role of the state as against the autonomy of the individual, whether constructed as 'citizen' or 'consumer', is critical in contemporary societies, and never more so than in public health, where the balance between a paternalist or 'nanny state' and neo-liberal consumerist freedom to value a collective good is under challenge throughout Europe and beyond. Authors in this volume largely propose a clear role for the state, both in addressing the determinants of health and in recognising and valuing changes in outcomes (what counts as success and who decides), and are wary of policy options that shift responsibility on to individuals. Each of these is elaborated below, with a final concluding section on future challenges.

## Inequalities: health, income and wealth

Authors use the perspective of their different disciplinary approaches to engage with contemporary debates on relative and absolute inequalities and causal explanations. Nick Spencer and Catherine Law (Chapter Five), in reviewing the impact of policy interventions on health inequalities experienced during pregnancy and early childhood, conclude that, despite numerous initiatives, such inequalities will not be reduced without further structural changes. In the field of diet and nutrition (Chapter Eight), where inequality gradients have not been much addressed, Elizabeth Dowler and her colleagues discuss the interpretation of outcome data in relation to various indicators of relative socioeconomic deprivation operating at both individual or household and geographic area levels, and consider the implications for policy intervention. However, they also provide evidence of absolute poverty in referring to research that demonstrates that, notwithstanding people's actual choices of expenditure, the money available to those who live in contemporary Britain on state means-tested benefits, pensions, or the minimum wage is insufficient to sustain healthy living, defined according to current guidelines and realistically costed. Hannah Bradby and Tarani Chandola (Chapter Six) point up the ways in which racism and discrimination compound the experience of poverty, particularly in terms of structural disadvantage. They argue that 'ethnicity, like class and gender, is a complex, dynamic and contingent characteristic whose properties can pertain to individuals, families and larger groups' (p 106).

The capacity for epidemiological research to capture these complexities, as in the practice of 'food choice', meaning of 'home', or understanding of 'class', is limited, as discussed in Chapters Eight, Seven and Four, respectively. Chapters Four and Eight, in reflecting on the theoretical underpinnings of understanding inequalities, thus draw attention to sociology's contribution to fleshing out, or even challenging, the numbers games (or 'political arithmetic', as Murcott, 2002, put it). This echoes Nguyen and Peschard's call, not untypical of social science comment, to avoid 'methodological individualism, assumed universalism, and unidirectional causation' (Nguyen and Peschard, 2003, p 447), and to understand the 'ways in which those who are less well off trade in their long-term health for short-term gain': health is not always the priority that researchers or health professionals would have it (see Chapter Eleven). Furthermore, as Chapters Four and Five maintain, the progressive balance between 'risk' and 'protective' factors throughout the life cycle contributes fundamentally to both the so-called behavioural elements and structural determinants of health outcomes.

These issues of relative versus absolute inequalities, and of understanding causations, are critical in shaping intervention. Should health and social policy on inequalities concentrate on the poorest, or is a whole-population focus needed? Ray Earwicker (Chapter Two) puts the current government view, that elevating health inequalities to an NHS priority has enabled the designation of the most deprived local authority areas as the 'spearhead' groups for action including 'seeking out and sharing good practice' (p 29; DH, 2006). Shaw and colleagues (2005) argue elsewhere that redistributive measures, addressing wealth even more than income inequalities, are essential to reduce inequalities in health: 'spearhead' focus will not work. Broadly, this is the line taken in Chapters Five and Eleven; other authors similarly endorse population focus within their speciality, rather than targeting specific groups or areas designated as needy. Nonetheless, we should not lose sight of the critical issue raised in Chapter Eight mentioned earlier, that levels of income for people who have to live on the minimum wage or state-administered benefits should be sufficient to enable healthy living. While this framing is a reductionist one, and leads to debate as to how the state should determine appropriate income levels, its importance here is in reminding us that, even in rich nations like the UK, there are families and individuals whose circumstances and experiences are of poverty and deprivation because of insufficient money, with all the concomitant problems that engenders (many of which are documented in this volume). This issue is seldom addressed in health inequalities policy rhetoric, and, as Dowler and colleagues comment (see p 138), was explicitly excluded by the previous Conservative government in constructing terms of reference for the Low Income and Diet Project Team. Despite representation to the current Prime Minister on the topic (for example, Zacchaeus 2000 Trust, 2004), it remains off the agenda.

Most contributors to this volume argue that, while simply enabling the poorest to have sufficient money might be seen as naive or insufficient as a solution, addressing inequalities in both income and wealth nonetheless carries a weight of evidence of likely impact. The political dimension both to raising the incomes of the poorest and to reducing inequalities is rather less familiar territory in the health inequalities literature (Chapter Three; Stewart-Brown, 2000). Stewart-Brown argues that, looking purely at UK income distribution, inequalities reduction would be more readily achieved by reducing income in the highest decile than increasing that of the lowest; Shaw et al (2005) would include wealth redistribution as well. Changes in the tax and benefits system, along with poverty reduction programmes under New Labour, have partially succeeded in reducing child poverty, unemployment and some measures of income inequality (Spencer and Law, Chapter Five, this volume; Sutherland et al, 2003; Evans and Scarborough, 2006; Seager, 2006). However, the interventions largely depend on paid work as a route out of poverty, which some argue demeans parental and other caring responsibilities, and often presents its own problems of sustainability and actual levels of living (Chapter Eleven; Payne, 2006). And, measurement complexities and details of effects notwithstanding (Jones, 2006), they have not reversed the huge disparities of the 1980s, when market liberalisation, an increase in property values and wage rises contributed to an unprecedented and still untouched increase in income and wealth inequalities (Chapter Three; Hills, 1998; Hills and Stewart, 2005). These factors are critical in contributing to the continuing health inequalities (Chapters Three and Five; Palmer et al, 2006). Reduction in adverse psychosocial environments may contribute to reducing inequalities, which may be behind the current endorsement in *Choosing health* of publicly funded therapists to reduce 'personal and social malaise' (Moloney, 2006), but this strategy is unlikely to succeed if the fundamental capitalist drivers of inequality, or, as Simon Williams and colleagues in Chapter Four put it, 'the readiness or willingness, let alone the ability in the global era, to take on entrenched powerful corporate interests whose prime concern is the making of healthy profits rather than healthy people' (p 62) are ignored.

Evidence cited on general morbidity and mortality by ethnic group, and in relation to housing, diet and obesity, all shows that, despite implementation of some 'upstream' interventions, outcome inequalities persist and, in some cases, are widening. Furthermore, there are categories of 'new poor' whose health is likely to contribute to inequality statistics, where targeted intervention is the strategy, but is piecemeal and as yet not wholly successful. These categories include asylum seekers, Traveller/Roma communities and the homeless/roofless (Chapters Six, Ten and Twelve). These chapters, along with Chapters Eight and Eleven, also elaborate the difficulties of 'targeting', both by characteristic such as minority ethnic status, or by area, age or some other deprivation proxy indicator. Indeed, the political usefulness of inequality-based targets is discussed from different perspectives, in Chapter Two as a means of engendering and maintaining political engagement across sectors, and in Chapter Three as a means of monitoring political aims and achievements. Garnering political support for meeting the needs of specific groups by differential intervention can itself be challenging: preventing 'children' from suffering has considerable salience, but some argue that even the reasonably successful achievements in reducing child poverty in the UK are played down and insufficiently promoted (Toynbee, 2006). What hope, then, of raising the profile of older unemployed men or asylum seekers as being also in need, whether on the grounds of reducing costs to the economy or NHS (the basis on which Wanless (2002, 2004) argues) or on grounds of social justice?

## What can governments do: what has the government done?

Marmot and his colleagues, in reviewing policies implemented following the Acheson Inquiry, concluded that 'there is much activity that is likely to have a favourable impact on health inequalities' (Marmot, 2004b, p 263) but that whether or not these actions would lead to a reduction in inequalities would need monitoring until 2010 and beyond (see also Chapter Five in this volume). That there was considerable cross-cutting activity, as well as efforts to bring coherence to initial disparate projects and funding initiatives, is attested throughout this volume as elsewhere (Exworthy et al, 2003). More critically, many departments and sectors hitherto unconcerned with 'health' and in some cases, with 'inequalities' found themselves engaging in a national project to tackle them, both in the aftermath of the Acheson Inquiry (Chapter Two) and through the powerful 'cross-cutting' spending reviews conducted by Sir Derek Wanless for the Treasury (Wanless, 2002, 2004).

New Labour's 'Third Way' tried to steer between leaving all to the state or all to individuals' responses to the private sector, and has led to varied attempts at partnership working, both between public sectors, including health, social care, local government and planning, and between the public sector and the private sector. The realities of 'joined-up solutions to joined-up problems' (p 178 in Chapter Ten) are examined in Chapters Eight, Ten, Eleven and Twelve). Most argue that a major failing has been the drift to 'projectisation', with a lack of sufficient investment of resources, training and ongoing support. Another has been the demand for rapid results in terms of outcomes set from above, with little real engagement with locally expressed needs and hopes about ill health and health – either in terms of intervention, or of desired and thus monitored/evaluated outcomes – whether this is characterised as 'user involvement', 'lay knowledge' or 'local empowerment'. However, Chapter Twelve gives examples from within social work's remit where some imaginative, collaborative efforts have produced practical support that contributes incrementally to reducing health inequalities: 'tweaking' the system, one might say, though apparently to good effect. David Ormandy's account (Chapter Seven) of developments in housing standards assessment highlights both that current policy has gone further than the general Acheson recommendations and that the driving force has in fact largely been outside the public health sector. He also draws attention to the potentially strong opportunities for collaborative action on housing between health and local government, and argues that this would both contribute to reducing health inequalities and fulfil environmental demands over energy use (WHO, 2005).

Ironically, in a period when targets and objectives have increasingly been set from the centre, *Choosing health* claims to be the result of devolving the power to shape policy to the people: 'it is the public who have, for the first time, set the agenda and identified what "for their own good" means, not Whitehall' (DH, 2004, p2), a claim that is examined here by several authors. 'Choice' has thus become the rhetoric of individual responsibility in both senses: recognising autonomy and ascribing culpability. The current personalisation focus limits state intervention in order to protect people's autonomy, under the explicit assumptions that people choose their 'lifestyle' and simply need help to realise personal goals (and perhaps motivation to improve them). Should they not do so, people have only themselves to blame: the state is not responsible (Food Ethics Council, 2005). The limitations of these views are exposed in Chapters Three, Four, Five, Eight and Eleven. Even the consultation process that preceded the White Paper demonstrated that the public recognised the complexities of the matter: while a large majority agreed that individuals are primarily responsible for their own health, 60% thought tackling poverty would be the most effective way of preventing illness and 40% (more in lower socioeconomic groups) felt there were 'too many factors outside individual control to hold people responsible for their own health' (DH, 2004; Opinion Leader Research, 2004).

The framing in terms of consumer choice is important: people constructed as 'consumers' rather than, say, citizens, voters, patients or users (see Chapter Ten) can lead to conflation of a political concept with an economic one, to the detriment of citizenship (Gabriel and Lang, 2006). The consumer as an individual economic agent making personal choices in a marketplace (in this instance, for health 'behaviour' inputs) is a misrepresentation and over-simplification of a reality in which, for most people living in areas of deprivation and/or on low incomes, 'choice' is constrained by structural and external factors, or by expectations and immediate life demands (as discussed in Chapters Four, Eight, Nine, Ten and Eleven). Furthermore, people do not on the whole operate as individual economic actors, even over 'health behaviour'; for instance, the decision to smoke or eat certain foods is governed by social norms and practices, even more so the management of wider determinants of health. This surely has resonance for a government anxious to engage with its public over health improvement, rather than dictate the means of achieving well-being.

Constructing the public as heterogeneous citizens recognises them as members of overlapping communities and networks of loyalties and communication, in which beliefs, attitudes and practices revolve and mesh in complex ways to demonstrate 'lifestyle' decisions. By contrast, the use of social marketing techniques to engage with people in provision of information/motivation for behavioural change presupposes that change at the individual level is the major need, and that mimicking the marketplace is the way to achieve it (see Chapters Four, Five, Eight, Ten and Eleven). As Hunter argues (2005, p 1011) public health thus faces a dilemma 'as by definition its work is carried out in the public realm and lies outside a market framework'. Rayner, a heart health promotion specialist who has tested the so-called 'traffic light' front of food package labelling for the UK Food Standards Agency, similarly points out that health-related behaviour is neither voluntary nor a product to be 'sold' (Rayner, 2006). The driving forces on health are increasingly located at regional, national and global levels, and need parallel governance responses (Beaglehole and Bonita, 2003).

One further common area of discussion is the role that information plays in government policy making, both in problem definition (discussed in Chapters Three, Seven and Eight) and in monitoring and evaluating outcomes or fine tuning intervention. The idea that policy operates within a rational, simple loop model of problem definition, selection of priorities, construction of targets and interventions, with monitoring and evaluation contributing to a feedback loop, has long been contested (Hogwood and Gunn, 1984). Evidence from research and information from monitoring and surveillance are probably used in more complex and subtle ways than a simple problem-solving model might imply (Berridge and Thom, 1996), as Elliot and Popay (2000) illustrate in their examination of how policy making was carried out by local health authorities in the UK. Chapter Ten in particular discusses the ways in which the voice of those characterised as 'users' is, or is not, taken into account, and as already mentioned, several contributors point to the distinction between outcomes desired by policy makers and those of the general public. The roles of different professionals and sectoral groups working together, and their differential power relationships, as well as the part played by civil society in the policy-making process, are discussed in Chapters Seven to Twelve; it is a striking common theme.

## Future challenges

Clearly, determinants of health operate at many levels, and need concomitant policy response. However, governance issues become even more challenging when devolved nation governments, as well as those at regional and international level, come into play. The UK presidency of the EU led to policy review of health inequalities, which in turn generated reviews of approaches and actions by different member states (Judge et al, 2006; Mackenbach, 2006; see also Whitehead, 1998 for an earlier example). In terms of devolved nations, a recent independent evaluation of 10 years of the Scottish Diet Action Plan (Lang et al, 2006) grappled with layered governance issues over food – which itself exemplifies much of the foregoing discussion: individuals choose what to eat, but multinational corporations grow/ship/process and retail it, with governments at various levels trying to regulate and facilitate 'healthy' choice. In the evaluation, the role of civil society and public opinion/public pressure in driving public health policy change was highlighted by expert witnesses in a number of areas: tobacco and health[1], school meals policy[2] and in Scottish legislation on protecting the right to feed an infant (effectively, to breastfeed) in public.[3] The evaluation of Scottish food and nutrition policy also linked the public health agenda to a wider framework of sustainability and environmental justice. Policy goals that cut across and link traditional sectors to sustainable development and social justice raise questions – in this instance, across the food system – that are broader than the usual public health policies (for example, simply encouraging people to 'eat five portions of fruit and vegetables a day' or to 'eat a balanced diet'). Government 'room to manoeuvre' in changing the focus and behaviour of important economic players (in this instance, food producers, importers, processors, manufacturers, distributors, retailers and caterers) is circumscribed by both private sector power and regulation by the EU and World Trade Organization. Nevertheless, public health's insistence on good health for all can be a powerful voice advocating 'for sustained political will and for government's stewardship role to be championed both within nation states and increasingly between them' (Hunter, 2005, p 1011).

Public health policy concerned with health inequalities thus should not focus only on those who experience the effects of health inequalities, but on all of society. It should engage with social justice: who cares whether or not inequalities are worsening or improving? The consequence of locating problems at the individual level is, as argued earlier, that culpability is located there too: if poor people's health does not improve, it is their own fault. And all too easily they too bear the responsibility in the other sense – of effecting improvement. The authors of this volume eschew such an outcome: responsibility in both senses belongs to the whole of society, and to different professions and disciplines within it, whether or not 'health outcomes' are traditionally or solely their business. These authors have contributed largely in the hope of generating interest both in and within disciplinary perspectives not often heard in the health inequalities debate, and to point to innovative work as well as professional and personal challenges to achieving the desired outcomes.

However, one fundamental challenge to all of us working in these fields is the emerging international evidence of new drivers of inequalities in climate change, sustainability of oil and water supply and globalisation's effects on many of the social determinants of health and healthcare provision. The health impacts of such factors were not widely understood a decade ago, were not on the New Labour agenda when it was elected and were thus outside the remit of the Acheson Inquiry, to which much of this book relates. This perception is shifting within the political field and to some extent in research,[4] where they are being raised in the context of environmental justice and inequalities (Walker and Eames, 2006). In its broadest terms, this is an international agenda, but one that links strongly to a national or rich nation debate. Climate change is now clearly on the political agenda in the UK as elsewhere; inequalities are much less highlighted within the debate, including the implications for health. Every issue discussed in this volume will be made worse if climate change and environmental degradation continue as at present; the inclusion of health impact assessments within other sustainability audits could at least make such undesirable results explicit. Recent work from the Sustainable Consumption Round Table explores the seeming paradox that high levels of economic growth have not led to corresponding improvements in well-being (Jackson, 2005) and looks at ways to engender wider acceptance and practice of the proposal that better and more equitable and sustainable living would be possible if consumption were reduced. This proposal works for public health as well: a consumerist approach will not work, particularly for reducing inequalities; the pursuit of social justice has great potential to be better for health and ensure happiness for all.

## Notes

[1, 2] www.scotland.gov.uk (for school meals, search on 'Hungry for Success').

[3] www.opsi.gov.uk/legislation/scotland/acts2005/20050001.htm

[4] For example, the Economic and Social Research Council/Natural Environment Research Council programme, Inequality and Sustainable Consumption.

# References

Acheson, D. (1998) *Independent inquiry into inequalities in health*, London: The Stationery Office.

Adams, J., White, M., Moffat, S., Howel, D. and Mackintosh, J. (2006) 'A systematic review of the health, social and financial impacts of welfare rights advice delivered in healthcare settings', *BMC Public Health*, vol 6, p 81 (www.biomedcentral.com/1471-2458/6/81).

Asthana, S. and Halliday, J. (2006) *What works in tackling health inequalities? Pathways, policies and practice through the lifecourse*, Bristol: The Policy Press.

Beaglehole, R. and Bonita, R. (2003) 'Strengthening public health for the new era', in R. Beaglehole (ed) *Global public health: A new era*, Oxford: Oxford University Press.

Berridge, V. and Thom, B. (1996) 'Research and policy: what determines the relationship?', *Policy Studies*, vol 17, no 1, pp 23-34.

Dahl, E., Fritzell, J., Lahelma, E., Martikainen, P., Kunst, A. and Mackenbach, J.P. (2006) 'Welfare state regimes and health inequalities', in S. Siegrist and M. Marmot (eds) *Social inequalities in health: New evidence and policy implications*, Oxford: Oxford University Press.

Davey Smith, G. (ed) (2003) *Health inequalities: Lifecourse approaches*, Bristol: The Policy Press.

DH (Department of Health) (1999) *Saving lives: Our healthier nation*, Cm 4386, London: The Stationery Office.

DH (2004) *Choosing health: Making healthier choices easier*, Cm 6374, London: The Stationery Office.

DH (2006) *Health challenge England: Next steps for 'Choosing health'*, London: DH.

Elliott, H. and Popay, J. (2000) 'How are policy makers using evidence? Models of research utilisation and local NHS policy making', *Journal of Epidemiology and Community Health*, vol 54, no 6, pp 461-8.

Emberson, J.R., Whincup, P.H., Morris, R.W. and Walker, M. (2004) 'Reducing social inequalities and the prevention of coronary heart disease', *International Journal of Epidemiology*, vol 33, no 5, pp 1152-3.

Evans, M. and Scarborough, J. (2006) *Can current policy end child poverty in Britain by 2020?*, York: Joseph Rowntree Foundation.

Exworthy, M., Stuart, M., Blane, D. and Marmot, D. (2003) 'Tackling health inequalities since the Acheson Inquiry', *Findings*, March 2003, York: Joseph Rowntree Foundation (www.jrf.org.uk).

Food Ethics Council (2005) *Getting personal: Shifting responsibilities for dietary health*, Brighton: Food Ethics Council (http://foodethicscouncil. org).

Gabriel, Y. and Lang, T. (2006) *The unmanageable consumer: Contemporary consumption and its fragmentation* (2nd edn), London: Sage Publications.

Graham, H. and Kelly, M. (2004) *Health inequalities: Concepts, frameworks and policy*, Briefing Paper, London: Health Development Agency.

Hills, J. (1998) *Income and wealth: The latest evidence*, York: Joseph Rowntree Foundation.

Hills, J. and Stewart, K. (eds) (2005) *A more equal society? New Labour, poverty, inequality and exclusion*, Bristol: The Policy Press.

Hogwood, B.W. and Gunn, L.A. (1984) *Policy analysis for the real world*, Oxford: Oxford University Press.

Hunter, D.J. (2005) 'Choosing or losing health?', *Journal of Epidemiology and Community Health*, vol 59, no 12, pp 1010-13.

Jackson, T. (2005) 'Live better by consuming less?', *Journal of Industrial Ecology*, vol 9, nos 1-2, pp 19-36.

Jones, F. (2006) 'The effects of taxes and benefits on household income, 2004/05', *Economic Trends 630*, Office for National Statistics, May, pp 53-70.

Judge, K., Platt, S., Costongs, C. and Jurczak, K. (2006) *Health inequalities: A challenge for Europe*, Independent expert report commissioned and published by the UK Presidency of the EU, London: Department of Health.

Lang, T., Dowler, E. and Hunter, D. (2006) *Review of the Scottish Diet Action Plan: Progress and impacts 1996–2005*, Edinburgh: NHS Health Scotland (www.healthscotland.com/understanding/evaluation/policy-reviews/review-diet-action.aspx).

Lang, T., Rayner, G. and Kaelin, E. (2006) *The food industry, diet, physical activity and health: A review of reported commitments and practice of 25 of the world's largest food companies*, London: City University.

Lynch, J., Davey Smith, G., Harper, S. and Bainbridge, K. (2006) 'Explaining the social gradient in coronary heart disease: comparing relative and absolute risk approaches', *Journal of Epidemiology and Community Health*, vol 60, no 5, pp 436-41.

Mackenbach, J. (2006) *Health inequalities: Europe in profile*, Independent expert paper commissioned and published by the UK Presidency of the EU. London: Department of Health.

Marmot, M. (2004a) 'Commentary: risk factors or social causes?', *International Journal of Epidemiology*, vol 33, no 2, pp 297-8.

Marmot, M. (2004b) 'Tackling health inequalities since the Acheson Inquiry', *Journal of Epidemiology and Community Health*, vol 58, no 4, pp 262-3.

Moloney, P. (2006) 'Unhappiness is inevitable', *The Guardian*, 28 August.

Morgan, K. (2006) 'School food and the public domain: the politics of the public plate', *The Political Quarterly*, vol 77, no 3, pp 379-87.

Murcott, A. (2002) 'Nutrition and inequalities: a note on sociological approaches', *European Journal of Public Health*, vol 12, no 3, pp 203-7.

Nguyen, V.-K. and Peschard, K. (2003) 'Anthropology, inequality, and disease: a review', *Annual Review of Anthropology*, vol 32, pp 447-74 (abstract at http://arjournals.annualreviews.org/doi/abs/10.1146/annurev.anthro.32.061002.093412?journalCode=anthro, accessed 24 August 2006).

Opinion Leader Research (2004) *Public attitudes to public health policy, summary*, London: King's Fund.

Palmer, G., Carr, J. and Kenway, P. (2006) *Monitoring poverty and social exclusion 2006*, York: Joseph Rowntree Foundation (www.jrf.org.uk; report on Scotland and Wales available from same site or www.poverty.org.uk).

Payne, L. with Fisher, H. (2006) *Unequal choices: Voices of experience exposing challenges and suggesting solutions to ending child poverty in the UK*, London: End Child Poverty in association with Joseph Rowntree Foundation.

Rayner, M. (2006) 'Could techniques that sell "unhealthy" food be used to market health instead?', *Food Ethics Council Bulletin*, vol 1, no 2, p 10 (www.foodethicscouncil.org).

Seager, A. (2006) 'Average income of richest 20% is 16 times that of the poorest', *The Guardian*, 13 May.

Shaw, M., Davey Smith, G. and Dorling, D. (2005) 'Health inequalities and New Labour: how the promises compare with real progress', *BMJ*, vol 330, pp 1016-21.

Stewart-Brown, S. (2000) 'What causes social inequalities: why is this question taboo?', *Critical Public Health*, vol 10, no 2, pp 233-42.

Sutherland, H., Sefton, T. and Piachaud, D. (2003) *Poverty in Britain: The impact of government policy since 1997*, York: Joseph Rowntree Foundation.

Thorogood, M., Simera, I., Dowler, E., Summerbell, C. and Brunner, B. (2007) 'A systematic review of population and community dietary interventions to prevent cancer', *Nutrition Research Reviews*, vol 20, no 1, pp 75-89.

Toynbee, P. (2006) 'We will never abolish child poverty in a society shaped like this one', *The Guardian*, 7 July.

WHO (World Health Organization) (2005) *Fourth Ministerial Conference on Environment and Health. Final report*, Copenhagen: WHO Regional Office for Europe.

Walker, G. and Eames, M. (2006) *Environmental inequalities*, Cross-cutting themes for the ESRC/NERC Transdisciplinary Seminar Series on Environmental Inequalities 2006-08 (available from www.sd-research. org.uk/events/documents/EIseminarsdiscussionpaperrevised.pdf or www.sd-research.org.uk/events/Seminars.php).

Wanless, D. (2002) *Securing our future health: Taking a long-term view. Final report*, London: HM Treasury (www.hm-treasury.gov.uk/consultations_and_legislation/wanless/consult_wanless_final.cfm).

Wanless, D. (2004) *Securing good health for the whole population. Final report*, London: HM Treasury (www.hm-treasury.gov.uk/consultations_and_legislation/wanless/consult_wanless04_final.cfm).

Watts, R., McGlone, P., Russell, J., Tull, K. and Dowler, E. (2006) 'Establishing, implementing and maintaining a social support infant feeding programme', *Public Health Nutrition*, vol 9, no 6, pp 714-21.

Whitehead, M. (1998) 'Diffusion of ideas on social inequalities in health: a European perspective', *The Milbank Quarterly*, vol 76, no 3, pp 469-92.

Zacchaeus 2000 Trust (2004) *Memorandum to the Prime Minister on minimum income standards*, London: Zacchaeus 2000 Trust.

# Index

Page references for notes are followed by n

## Health inequalities and welfare resources
### Continuity and change in Sweden
*Edited by **Johan Fritzell** and **Olle Lundberg***

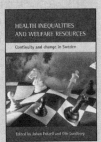

How welfare states influence population health and health inequalities has long been debated but less well tested by empirical research. This book presents new empirical evidence of the effects of Swedish welfare state structures and policies on the lives of Swedish citizens. However, the discussion, analysis and innovative theoretical approaches developed in the book have wide implications for health research and policy beyond Scandinavian borders.

**PB** £24.99 US$39.95 **ISBN** 978 1 86134 757 2
**HB** £55.00 US$90.00 **ISBN** 978 1 86134 758 9
240 x 172mm 264 pages December 2006 Health and Society Series

## Community health and well-being
### Action research on health inequalities
*Edited by **Steve Cropper, Alison Porter, Gareth Williams, Sandra Carlisle, Robert S Moore, Martin O'Neill, Chris Roberts** and **Helen Snooks***

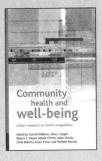

This book argues that the traditional government approach of exhorting individuals to live healthier lifestyles is not enough – action to promote public health needs to take place not just through public agencies, but also by engaging community assets and resources in their broadest sense. We need to be bolder in our approaches to community-based health improvement and more flexible in our understanding of the ways in which knowledge informs developments in health policy.

**PB** £19.99 US$36.95 **ISBN** 978 1 86134 818 0
**HB** £65.00 US$99.00 **ISBN** 978 1 86134 819 7
234 x 156mm 248 pages tbc October 2007 Health and Society Series

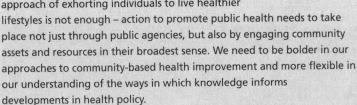

# The handbook of inequality and socioeconomic position
## Concepts and measures
*Mary Shaw, Bruna Galobardes, Debbie A. Lawlor, John Lynch, Ben Wheeler* and *George Davey Smith*

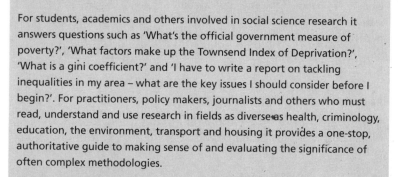

This handbook is the definitive resource for anyone wishing to quickly look up and understand key concepts and measurements relating to socioeconomic position and inequalities.

For students, academics and others involved in social science research it answers questions such as 'What's the official government measure of poverty?', 'What factors make up the Townsend Index of Deprivation?', 'What is a gini coefficient?' and 'I have to write a report on tackling inequalities in my area – what are the key issues I should consider before I begin?'. For practitioners, policy makers, journalists and others who must read, understand and use research in fields as diverse as health, criminology, education, the environment, transport and housing it provides a one-stop, authoritative guide to making sense of and evaluating the significance of often complex methodologies.

**PB** £19.99 US$35.00 **ISBN** 978 1 86134 766 4
**HB** £55.00 US$90.00 **ISBN** 978 1 86134 767 1
240 x 172mm 248 pages June 2007 Health and Society Series

To order copies of these publications or any other Policy Press titles please visit **www.policypress.org.uk** or contact:

**In the UK and Europe:**
Marston Book Services, PO Box 269,
Abingdon, Oxon, OX14 4YN, UK
Tel: +44 (0)1235 465500
Fax: +44 (0)1235 465556
Email: direct.orders@marston.co.uk

**In the USA and Canada:**
ISBS, 920 NE 58th Street, Suite 300,
Portland, OR 97213-3786, USA
Tel: +1 800 944 6190
(toll free)
Fax: +1 503 280 8832
Email: info@isbs.com

**In Australia and
New Zealand:**
DA Information Services,
648 Whitehorse Road Mitcham,
Victoria 3132, Australia
Tel: +61 (3) 9210 7777
Fax: +61 (3) 9210 7788
E-mail: service@dadirect.com.au